MORE PRAISE FOR
EVOLVE: FOCUS ON FITNESS

"John's book got us motivated to stop making excuses and start living a healthy lifestyle...thanks to John we have begun exercising together as a family and we have never looked or felt better! Thanks John!"

Jen and Steven Wakser
Busy Parents of 3 Children

"John got me excited about getting fit. He motivated me by not only telling me I could accomplish anything but by teaching me how to. He tells you the truth about fitness and lifestyle change. John helped me change from a 28% body fat blob into a 10% body fat rock-solid man in 3 months. That lifestyle change unleashed the real me. And most importantly, that lifestyle change, influenced me in mind, body, and spirit."

Ron Chambers
Fitness Professional

"John's honesty is refreshing. By following the Focus on Fitness program I've seen results I never dreamed possible."

Cathy Carmany
Banking Executive

"John's step-by-step approach makes it easy to not only lose fat, but to get fit while your doing it."

Mike Ficzner
Lieutenant US Army
Black Hawk Platoon Leader

"What makes this book different than all the other weight loss and exercise books on the market right now is that this one really works!"

Louis J. Berrodin
Financial Planner

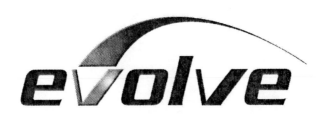

FOCUS ON FITNESS:

THE TRUTH ABOUT FAT, FADS, & FITNESS

JOHN COOK

FITNESS PRESS

ISBN: 1-59268-053-4

Fitness Press
New York, New York
A Division of GMA Publishing

Check out our website.
GMA is a global publishing company
Our books are available and distributed around the world and can be found on
the internet at Amazon, Barnes and Noble and any major bookseller.

GMAPublishing@aol.com
GMAPublishing.com

Cover By: thunder::tech
Manuscript Design: thunder::tech
Manuscript Assistant: John Beanblossom
Photo Layout: thunder::tech
Inset Photography: King Louie Photo

thunder::tech is a marketing and advertising firm specializing in web, database,
and identity design. You can visit them on the web at thundertech.com.

Printed in the United States of America

It is strongly suggested that before beginning ANY exercise program or making dramatic
changes in your diet you should first consult your physician.

Also be advised that taking part in any physical activity can result in injury or even death. If
at any time you feel dizziness or nausea you should stop what your doing immediately and
rest. If you do not recover immediately, do not hesitate to contact your doctor.

You are taking part in this program of your own free will. Evolve Inc., assumes no respon-
sibility for injuries or illness that may occur during exercise.

The program outlined in this book is a very effective and proven method to becoming fit
the right way. In no way does it promise amazing results overnight. Only by making exercise and proper diet part of your lifestyle will you achieve your fitness goals.

DEDICATIONS

To my mother, Linda, who taught me the importance of building and developing a strong mind.

To my father, John, who taught me the importance of building a strong body.

To my wonderful wife, Tracy, who encouraged me to write this book and who has always supported me in my crusade to help people unlock their true (fitness) potential.

And mostly, I thank God, because without Him, I would be nothing.

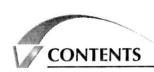

CONTENTS

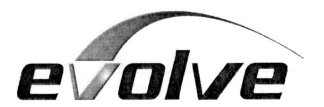

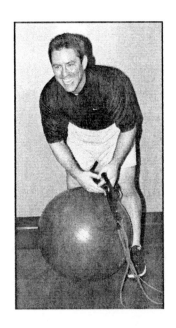

Happiness is Fitness.
-John Cook

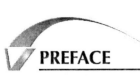

PREFACE

WHAT SETS MY MESSAGE APART

Evolve: (*verb*)   To change.

Fitness: (*noun*)   The ability to physically, mentally and emotionally deal with everyday environmental challenges.

Those who are fit deal with everyday challenges more effectively. Those who are unfit struggle with daily challenges.

Anyone can show you what to do to change, but the trick is to motivate you to change the way you think first. No matter how effective a program is, if you aren't motivated to do it, what good is it? This book will not only educate you on what to do but it will motivate you to do it!

This book was not written to teach you how to build a massive physique or have Hulk-like strength. It was not written to show you proper training to run a marathon or compete in a triathlon. It was not written to teach you how to bench press 300 pounds or squat 400 pounds. It was not written to teach you exercise physiology or kinesiology. It <u>was</u> written to motivate and teach you, in the simplest way, to transform your body into a healthy and fit one. It was written to help you realize that being fit is not a battle of muscle, but a battle of will. That being fit will improve the quality of everything you do. Fitness is not defined as an abdominal six-pack, a 300 pound bench press, or the ability to run a marathon. It is simply defined as being able to deal physically, mentally and emotionally with daily challenges. By teaching your body to push itself everyday during your work-outs for a short time, other everyday activities will become easier and less demanding, mentally and physically. Once you implement this program into your lifestyle you will see that you are able to function at a level you may never have dreamed possible. If looking great and feeling great is your goal, then this is the book for you. And I will promise you that by following through with my method, you will build the foundation necessary to accomplish greatness. And if greatness to you is a six-pack of abs, a 300+ bench press or winning a triathlon, then GO FOR IT!

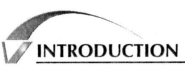

INTRODUCTION

YOU TOO CAN EVOLVE YOUR LIFE

My name is John Cook and I am just an ordinary guy that achieved extraordinary results by following a simple system I developed through lots of trial and error. I did this without the help of any professional fitness trainers, dieticians, nutritionists or emotional therapists. <u>You can do the same</u>. I know you can because many others like you that have failed countless times with fad programs, have followed my system and achieved unbelievable life changing results. You don't need to join a fancy health club or purchase a thousand dollar home gym. You surely don't need any wonder drinks or pills. Actually I strongly advise against it.

What you are about to read in this book will outline the blueprint for an extraordinary transformation of body, mind, and spirit. If you choose to follow these simple lifestyle suggestions, you will not only look better but you will feel younger,

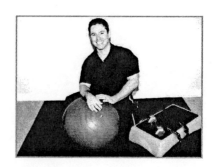

You only need a few inexpensive items and a positive attitude to have a really great workout!
-John Cook

sleep better and think at a level you never imagined possible. You will accomplish more than ever, deal with stress more efficiently and your interpersonal relationships will be dramatically enriched.

They say that different things work for different people, though this may be true, of all the people that had the courage to implement these basic lifestyle changes and take control of their lives, I have yet to see one fail, no matter what their genetic predisposition was at the beginning of the program. There is no fad diet involved or crazy exercise routine. Everything you need is obtainable at your local grocery store or in your home.

My system is based on how the human body was designed physiologically to be fed and exercised. After 14 days of following my program you will wish you had started sooner. You will achieve both a heightened mental clarity and physical confidence with your life.

There is NO excuse not to take action. You <u>can</u> do this and if you give it 100% you <u>will</u> do this. I cannot stress enough that this is possible. It is for real, I know, because I've seen it work. And it is not as hard as many of you may think. Persistence, planning, organization, and discipline are the keys. Not fad diets, creams, pills, crazy breathing techniques or ab gadgets! All you have to do is take one step towards change, one step to transforming you life forever. *Are you ready to evolve your life?*

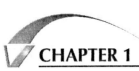

CHAPTER 1

MY STORY: THE TYPICAL AMERICAN LIFESTYLE

For the past several years, like most people (maybe even you), I have struggled with poor health. My exercise sessions were sporadic and my diet atrocious to say the least. Like most Americans I indulged in food and drink to my hearts content. It seemed that everything in my life revolved around eating and drinking. At every social event I attended there was a cocktail or beer offered to me, and comfort food was never too far behind.

I would have stretches where I would try a fad diet to lose the extra ten pounds I had put on over the winter months. Grapefruit diets, no-carb diet, liquid diet, no-eating diet, we know them all. Everyone says they've got a quick and easy way to shed the pounds while still enjoying the foods our bodies love so much. I took all the pills and drank all the drinks and followed all the programs only to be disappointed by the lack of lasting results. Many of us believe that just because it is advertised on TV or featured in a book or magazine it must be true, therefore, it must work! NOT SO! I remember seeing a commercial with all these "beautiful" people with ripped abs and perfect bodies lounging around a pool eating cheeseburgers, fried chicken and cake. We were supposed to believe that if you just took this carb-blocker you could eat like that, not exercise, and you would look like these models. I admit, for short moment I actually picked up the phone to order a lifetime supply! Then I came to my senses. If it was that easy, everyone would be doing it.

There are countless brilliant scientists out there working around the clock to develop products for businesses to market that claim to cut the fat. In reality, they really do little more than increase your trips to the bathroom. It is amazing to me that there are so many products available on the market that promise that just by taking a little pill you will look great and feel great. Why is it then that we continue to get fatter and fatter and our overall health gets more and more pitiful. When will we get wise to this nonsense?

I can remember trying the no-carb diet. Wow! That was the best thing going! I can eat steak, bacon, eggs and cheese all day and still lose weight. I did lose weight... and <u>fast</u>. But guess what? Most of it was water and I gained it all back plus more. Not to mention the horrendous effects it has on your body.

Several times I tried to do it correctly. I'd go to my local health club with the best intentions, only to find myself chatting for an hour and ending up in the sauna or steam room having accomplished nothing except a short walk on the treadmill or a couple sets of bicep curls. After my "work-outs" I'd have a false sense of accomplishment and I would treat myself to a 2000 calorie meal. Hey, I worked out today, I'll burn it off. If only then I realized how much exercise it takes to burn 2000 calories.

I never worried about the long-term effects of an unhealthy lifestyle because I was young and feeling great, I could eat what I wanted and not look "that" fat. But just because I did not "look" fat did not mean I wasn't terribly unhealthy.

At the young age of 30 I began to feel myself getting tired during the day for the first time. I would notice becoming out of breath after climbing a couple flights of stairs. After playing a pick-up game of basketball at the local YMCA it took me 3 days to recover from the soreness and burning in my muscles. Uh oh! I thought I was just getting older. That was my initial excuse. Even after I began to notice these changes in my fitness level I still continued to eat junk, drink too much, and neglect my body. What the heck, I had a good job, a great house and car and all the things I wanted, what could be better?

Then reality set in. I believe that once in everyone's life there is a life changing moment where an important decision has to be made. Life is full of choices. The way we handle these choices dictates the majority of what happens in our lives. Contrary to popular belief, I believe luck plays a very, very, small part. You get out what you put in, simple as that. The harder you work and the more you plan, the luckier you get. My life-changing moment was actually a chain of moments that really woke me up.

First, I was at my local bank making a deposit. A woman that I worked with a year before approached me to say "hi." I was always very friendly with this woman and she was the type to tell it like it was. After a few brief moments of chit-chat she commented to me that I had taken on a lot of weight. I immediately became defensive and said that my home and work responsibilities were taking up so much of my time there was none left to exercise. She smiled and said she understood and she hoped to see me again soon. I didn't think anything of it.

Later that evening I was visiting my aunt and uncle. After some small talk with my uncle, being the blunt individual he is, he looked at me and told me I was fat. WHAT! I said, "I'm getting fat?" He replied, "No, you <u>are</u> fat!" Immediately I became defensive again. I wasn't fat; I was just a little chubby. What did he know anyway? This is a guy that orders a bucket of fried chicken and just eats the skin! Yuck! I again used the same excuse as before. Stress, work, no time...<u>nonsense</u>! That night all I could think about was what happened during the day.

The next morning I awoke without a thought of what my uncle had said. Distracted by my daily responsibilities and stresses I made my way to work and started my day out as I usually did with a plate of corned beef hash and eggs and a couple cups of coffee. Little did I know that in a few hours my life would begin to change forever.

On my way home from work I stopped by the local drug store to pick-up some pictures I dropped off to be developed. I had to look at them as soon as they were handed to me and paid for. There's a good one of the dog… a cute one of the girlfriend…my best friend at a golf outing, then… OH MY GOSH! There I was in a bathing suit! Was that person really me? My love handles needed wheels. My gut was hanging over my suit and I was working on a second chin! What happened? I couldn't look like that. The bad news was, the picture was taken 10 pounds ago! I'm a *fat guy!*

All the energy was drained from my body. I felt a strange urge to hit the local pub and drown my sorrow in a 64 oz. beer and a giant order of chili cheese fries. This is where that choice thing comes into play. I went right back into the drug store and bought every fitness, health and bodybuilding magazine they had, drove straight home and began to feverishly thumb through each publication. As I skimmed my way through the first five or six I began to notice one very popular trend. Each magazine was filled with ad after ad for products that guaranteed an "amazing" transformation. You've surely seen them.

It was the same as before. Take this pill and go from a fat guy to a muscle guy in 12 short weeks. Drink this supplement and you are sure to lose 15% of your body-fat in three months. I saw all the "before" and "after" photos and thought... yeah, right! It had to be trick photography. Either that or it had to take longer than 12 weeks to do that! I had to admit though, that they did intrigue my curiosity. I thought that if it was possible I could do it. Everything else would come second. This would be my priority, my passion and my goal. I was sick of being tired, fat, and lazy. I had tried it their way and failed miserably. It was time to do it the right way. It was time to do it my way.

I was ready to *evolve*. Little did I know that I was ready to embark on a life-changing journey that would take a mere 80 days. This journey would not only transform my body but it would also transform my mind, spirit and complete way of thinking.

In the following pages, you too will learn how to evolve yourself into a more fit, efficient, and happy person. It takes some work, but I promise it's easier than you think, and once you get started, the outcome is worth a thousand times the investment.

CHAPTER 2

FACTS AND FICTION

I am going to outline in the simplest of terms exactly what you must do from start to finish. I am going to give you tips and tricks to stay focused, and ways to prevent yourself from failing. I am not going to go into too much detail of why this or that works and this does not. Or why this food is better than another. I am not going to preach to you or complicate things with scientific explanation. I am not going to bore you with physiological Latin, or cushy motivational phrases. Well, maybe some. I am going to show you effective exercises that you can do without leaving your home! I am going to give it to you straight. I am going to tell you the truth about transformation. I cannot stress enough that this is an attainable goal for anybody. I never thought in a million years that I would be able to accomplish this and stick with it, but I did. And so can you. This is for real and it's not as hard or complicated as you may think. Persistence, planning, and a little organization and discipline are the keys. There are no health drinks, powdered supplements, pills or vibrating belts in this program. Just basic food and a little moving are all you need to finally reach you goals of becoming a fitter, happier person. I will also teach you how to implement this new lifestyle so you never waiver again.

THE ANCESTOR PRINCIPLE

Our ancestors from the not so distant past were incredibly fit and efficient people. They had no choice but to be fit. Those who were not did not make it in such a hostile environment for too long. They were incredibly strong and had great endurance. Their bodies were very efficient at storing body fat to use as energy later. It may have been days or even weeks before early man could indulge in a substantial meal. Because of this, our bodies naturally want to store body fat. That was great then. But now, as food has become more readily accessible and our lifestyles more sedentary, we eat more calories than we need and burn fewer than we should. This leads to over-storage of fat. We never need to burn it later because there is a constant supply of food to be eaten. This is evident in the majority of Americans today. Because our physiologies have remained the same, and we have become almost totally reliant on technology we continue to get fatter and fatter.

THE FOURTH BASIC NEED

When we were just getting started as a human race we had three basic needs to survive: food, clothing, and shelter. As we became more technologically advanced in the past 100 years, we have added a fourth need: exercise. Early humans did not have the luxury of driving to the grocery store, filling up their cart with boxes and bags of food and taking it home to throw in the microwave and then into their mouths. There were no fast food restaurants to drive up to when they felt hungry, or bored. As a matter of fact, our ancestors were hunters and gatherers. They ate small meals throughout the day, and as a result, their metabolisms ran smoothly and efficiently. Also, they had to <u>work</u> to get food, clothing and shelter. They expended valuable energy stalking and catching animals to eat, lots of energy. They expended energy tilling land and planting gardens. They built homes with brute strength and made clothes with their bare hands. How big of a house would you live in if you had to build it? How much fatty beef would you eat if you had to chase it for two days and then <u>maybe</u> you would have a successful kill, or maybe not! Our bodies are designed to be pushed to limits far greater than most of us will ever experience. Imagine having a Ferrari and only driving it around town in first gear at 20 miles an hour! That's how most of us live our lives. That stinks! I have been on both ends of the spectrum and I'll tell you, healthy and fit are much, much better.

THE GENETIC EXCUSE

We as humans are very different looking on the outside but as you may or may not know, we are quite similar on the inside. A minor change in our genetic strand makes us different, but physiologically our bodies work almost identically. Of course there is always an exception to every principle or rule, but the exceptions to this principle are quite rare. Yes, there may be that 1 person in 100,000 that no matter what he or she does will just appear overweight or sluggish. There are rare cases of people that have a disease or disorder that prevents this principle from working for them. But I feel very confident that you are not one of those people. I hear quite often now from people at my seminars or in conversation that they have trouble because they have a "slow" metabolism. This may be true now, but it has not always been slow. Those of you who have young children can attest to this being ridiculous. How many times has a four-year old worn you out and begged for more? We control our own metabolism. If we eat smaller meals more frequently throughout the day, exercise properly, drink lots of water and get enough rest our metabolism speeds up. If we eat two big meals a day and sit on the couch and watch TV all night our metabolism slows down... simple as that.

Our bodies are extremely adaptable. Actually we are about the most adaptable of all creatures on earth. We can eat just about anything and live just about anywhere without too much problem. Our bodies adapt to whatever we are doing. If we sit on our butts and eat pizza and chicken wings that is what we will crave. If we eat a healthy diet and exercise, that's what our body will crave. I want everyone right now to understand that our bodies are also very forgiving. We can abuse them with fatty foods and lack of exercise for years, and after a short time of proper nutrition and fitness, we can shape them back up in no time at all. Even if you are as much as 100 pounds overweight, by developing some discipline in your lifestyle you can lose that weight properly in less than one year. That may seem like a long time, but it may have taken you half a lifetime to get that way. Pretty fair trade-off if you ask me.

All you have to do is look around, maybe even just in the mirror, to see that Americans are getting fatter and fatter. That just solidifies my observations that the fad diets and schemes are not working. It is just so easy to give in to temptation. We no longer eat for energy, we eat for pleasure or because we are bored or stressed. We are bored and stressed because we don't exercise and we are too fat. Very few people are actually taking care of themselves by living a healthy lifestyle or making proper food choices. We are even seeing Type II or Adult Onset diabetes in young children. Type II is, in the majority of cases, attributed to obesity. Fat children will most likely grow into fat adults. Obesity has reached epidemic proportions and there is no relief in sight, it is just going to get worse.

I recently saw a statistic that showed that 15% of Americans eat a 100% diet of fast food! I can see where it is tough though. It tastes good, it's cheap, and it's quick, what else could you want. There are very intelligent people that work for these fast-food companies. It is bad enough that these people are working on developing the best tasting foods by adding more fat and salt, but then there are the advertisers that make you want it. The last thing we need is a triple bacon cheeseburger at 2 in the morning! They should call it a triple by-pass cheeseburger. By eating this way we are slowly committing suicide. I will be the first one to admit that it is tough to avoid the temptation but it is far from impossible. Any of us can do it if we make the choice to do so.

Insanity is when you continue to do the same things over and over again while expecting a different result. If we don't stop putting off a healthy lifestyle our quality of life is going to be agonizing when we get older.

I have found that there are four major problems the majority of Americans that fail to become fit have in common.

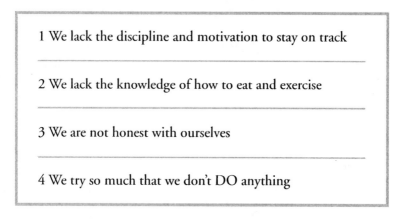

1 We lack the discipline and motivation to stay on track

2 We lack the knowledge of how to eat and exercise

3 We are not honest with ourselves

4 We try so much that we don't DO anything

DISCIPLINE AND MOTIVATION

Anything that requires discipline may be hard at first, but the long-term positive payoff is always much greater than the investment. Anything that is easy now may feel good for a short time, but most always has a short and then long-term negative repercussion. Think about it, anything you have ever done that took some work was always more rewarding than things that come easy. That trip to McDonald's sure seems like a good idea at the time but don't you feel like crap after you've indulged? And the long term effects are even scarier.

On the other hand, how many times have you worked out and felt like a million bucks when you were done? The trick is to <u>make</u> yourself do these positive things and before you know it they will become habit.

I will share with you over and over certain catch phrases to use everyday that will help you continue to be disciplined and motivated throughout this awesome journey. Those of you with the courage to take on these new challenges will enjoy healthy and happy lives!

THE VICIOUS DIET CYCLE

There is a simple way of explaining to people why they have failed in their attempts to lose weight. When someone begins a diet they instinctively lower their total caloric intake through starvation or fad dieting which usually includes cutting out a basic nutrient or consuming diet drinks and bars. Initially body weight falls. Most of the weight lost will be fluid stored in the body or food in the stomach and intestine.

Once our bodies realize that we have lowered our caloric intake it will naturally strive to maintain our original weight by becoming more energy efficient and slowing down our metabolism. At this point our bodies think we are <u>starving</u>! Feeling that it is starving, our bodies will begin to hold fat in order to survive, while learning to be more calorie efficient. In other words, our bodies begin to learn to function on fewer calories.

At this point, the body begins to search for other sources of fuel for energy. The first place it goes to find that energy, if we are not exercising, is muscle. The body is very good at deciding what it needs to exist. If we are not engaging in a resistance training program, the body senses that we do not need as much muscle as fat. The more muscle that is burned, the slower our metabolism becomes. Even if we stick to this, which only about 5% do, we are just becoming unfit, thin people.

After a short period, usually less than 21 days, the dieter will begin to experience a dramatic loss in energy, and will become tired and unfocused. In order to combat this, not only does the body start to crave sugar and fat, but more calories are ordered forcing us to binge on sweets and fat.

The worst part of this is seen when someone loses 10 pounds and gains 15 on this type of diet. This occurs because the body has learned to function on fewer calories. As soon as we increase our caloric intake again, these will be stored as fat. Whew!

THE CRISIS

60% of Americans are OVERFAT!

23 Million Women over age 20 are Obese (25%)

17 Million Men over age 20 are Obese (20%)

40 Million of Americans are Obese

10% of Americans are MORBIDLY OBESE!

1 in 3 American Children are OVERFAT!

(Only 5% 20 years ago!)

15% of Americans eat a 100% Fast Food Diet! YUCK!

25% of Americans are TOTALLY SEDENTARY!

75% of Americans are chronically dehydrated!

THE REASON

The reason we continue to fail is that we are focused on losing weight instead of getting fit! We worry so much about losing a couple pounds we don't focus on our fitness! Once you begin to become fit, the fat will disappear. As soon as you are able to understand

and believe this, you have half the battle won! We are a quick results oriented society. We want it now. So throughout the years, diet programs have focused on the idea of monitoring weight. This is totally absurd. There are many factors that come into play when it comes to losing weight.

Increased sodium intake, for instance, can hold a couple pounds of water in a single day. On the other hand decreasing your sodium intake can help reduce stored fluids in your system. Both of these factors can lead to a false sense of success or failure. So why are we still falling for these silly ideas and failure designed programs? Because we are so programmed to believe these lies are the truth. We see and hear them so much we actually start to believe they are true. I can't stand it when I see a success story of someone who has lost weight. They always say "I tried every program out there… and none of them worked!" It is not a program, it is a way of life. My program is a lifestyle commitment. Sensible diet and consistent exercise make people fit, not weight loss programs and magic juices or pills. From this point on, get ready to read about what really works, what really is the truth, get ready to EVOLVE YOUR LIFE..

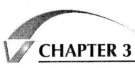

CHAPTER 3

GETTING INTO THE RIGHT STATE OF MIND

The first thing you need to do is forget everything you think is true about becoming fit and losing fat. There is <u>no</u> pill, there is <u>no</u> drink, there is <u>no</u> home abdominal machine, to make you fit. You may think I am being redundant, but why do we continue to fall for these lies? Fad Diets DO NOT WORK. There is no quick-fix. You must implement this as a LIFESTYLE.

The second thing you must realize is that with the proper tools and plans, we can build ourselves into whatever we want! If you don't invest in your body now, you will regret it terribly. You have to take action <u>now</u>! Do not put it off any longer.

REALIZE!

The hardest part is realizing that being unfit is a problem. Realize that there is a serious need to change, and understand that time is <u>now</u>! Realize that there are people that care about you. If you have children, or grandchildren, realize that they count on you to be there for them. Realize that they care about how you feel mentally and physically. Realize that investing in change now will pay you back 10 fold as you age. Realize that you must choose to change now, or have <u>no choice</u> but to change later. Realize that by then, it may be too late! Once you have conquered this, the rest will fall into place.

The longer you tell yourself you don't need to change or the longer you put off changing, or the longer you lie to yourself and make up excuses why you don't have time, the harder it becomes. Pick a day and start a new life. Once you pick that day, start and don't ever quit. You will not regret it, I PROMISE!

PRIORITIZE!

Get your priorities straight. As long as we continue to put everything before our health we will continue to be fat and unfit and our quality of life will suffer. The two excuses I hear most from people that are avoiding a fit lifestyle are: "I have no time." And "I am too tired." The reason people don't have time is their priorities are out of whack. These are the same people that sit in front of their computers for hours and surf the Internet or veg-out in front of the television for hours at a time. Television is <u>not</u> a priority! It numbs the brain. Use television as a reward you can give yourself after you have exercised.

Those that are "too tired" need to realize that they are tired because they are not exercising and eating right. By implementing a healthy lifestyle, not only will you learn to make time for exercise, but it will become a necessary part of your life. When you don't exercise your body will crave it and you won't feel right until you do it. The best thing about living a healthy lifestyle is that once your body begins to change, daily routines become easier, your energy levels increase dramatically, and you will naturally become more efficient. What all this leads to is being able to complete tasks more quickly, inevitably making more time for things that you enjoy.

The other excuse I hear from people that are avoiding living a healthy lifestyle is "I don't want to give up all the good stuff!" I ask them, "What do you mean by "the good stuff"?" It's always the same, sweets, fast food, chips, beer, cigarettes etc. Here's a news flash: THAT'S THE BAD STUFF!

VISUALIZE!

One of the easiest ways to achieve a goal is to physically close your eyes and imagine yourself doing what you dream of or looking like you dream you could look. If you are a salesperson, a great tool is to envision yourself closing a sale with that tough customer.

Professional athletes use this trick to imagine themselves doing the things they want to do, for example, hitting a baseball on the sweet-spot or swooshing that perfect basket. You should practice this with any goals you have. If you want to start your own business, close your eyes and picture yourself doing it! The same goes for achieving your fitness goals. If your goal is to look great, imagine yourself in that bikini on the beach or taking your shirt off at the pool and showing off that great new body. If your goal is to wear your jeans from high school or that dress you haven't put on since before you had kids, dare to imagine yourself in them! I promise this works.

Here is the best way to do it:

Sit or lay down in a comfortable room by

yourself where you know you will not be interrupted. If there is some music you like go ahead and play it, but I prefer absolute quiet. Begin to relax by closing your eyes and breathing slowly in through the nose, deeply and out through the mouth. Start to gently flex your entire body, starting with the toes and work your way up through your legs, back, neck and arms. Let all that daily stress leave your body. Begin to imagine yourself with that body you have always dreamed of. Keep your eyes closed until it is a very vivid picture.

Once you have come into focus, begin to breathe regularly concentrating on that mental image for a couple of minutes until it is planted in your memory. Imagine yourself actively doing things you wish you could do now (running, playing sports, climbing stairs with a spring in your step.) Imagine a pain-free life, imagine being stress-free, imagine feeling great!

Now slowly open your eyes, sit up and realize that what you just experienced is possible and that you CAN and WILL do it. If you follow the plan in this book, your present reality will be a memory, and your visualization will become reality.

ORGANIZE!

When I talk to people about why they have failed in the past they give me a multitude of interesting answers. "I couldn't stick with it," "It was too hard to eat 6 times a day." "I couldn't get my work-outs in with my busy schedule." Blah, Blah, Blah. These people, like most of us, failed to <u>organize</u>. You must organize your life.

Organization is the key to productivity. How many times have you searched for paperwork throughout the house that you need for your taxes or your new mortgage? How often have you searched for a tool when you needed to fix something around the house? How often have you looked for that important number around the office that seemed to be nowhere to be found? Every place has its thing and every thing has its place. If you follow this your life will run much more efficiently.

The same goes for living a healthy lifestyle. If you don't organize your fitness plan before you begin you will fail. The two most important components of living a healthy lifestyle are your exercise sessions and your nutrition. Make sure you understand that making this a main priority you make everything else in you life better.

Have a game plan before you get started. Organize your fitness and nutritional arsenal. Make sure you have work-out clothes clean and ready. If you must, lay them out for the week. Keep your work-out area clean and organize it to your needs. If you are jumping rope on Thursday, make sure you know where your jump rope is on Monday. If you use a heart-rate monitor during your cardio training, have it ready and in the same place everyday. If you have trouble preparing meals everyday, make enough food for the week on Sunday and freeze them in individual containers. All you have to do is pull out a container and throw it in the microwave and *voila!* You have your meal.

Keep bottled water and healthy snacks in a cooler in your car. In case you get hungry while you are driving by the 10 million fast food restaurants on your street you can curb that craving with a big bottle of water or a healthy snack. If I am going to a function that fattening foods are being served, I will bring my own food and eat it on the way, when I get there, I will take a taste of something so not to offend the host. Always plan your nutrition and work-outs a week in advance and you will be on your way to success!

Keep your journal in the same spot all the time. Keep your training shoes in the same place. I don't know how many times I have heard of people getting frustrated before a work-out and not going because they couldn't find their sneakers. I can't tell you the number of

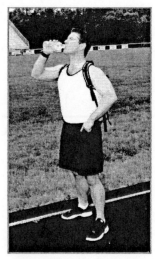

Drink plenty of water!

times clients have told me they had to eat at Wendy's because they were starving and had <u>no choice</u>!

Begin to organize your life, maintain the organization and you will see how things flow with ease. You will begin to accomplish things in a more timely fashion with more efficiency. Once you know where everything is, you will see that you have much more time than you need.

CHAPTER 4

BEFORE YOU GET STARTED

There are few easy things you need to do before you begin your journey. There is an old cliché that says, "If you fail to prepare, then prepare to fail." This is vital to achieving any goal but especially important when striving to achieve fitness goals. If you leave out any component, or fail to take any detail seriously, it will hinder your overall outcome.

Compare fitness to baking a cake (I know…I had to use cake). There are several components that go into baking a cake. You need flour, sugar, eggs etc. You also need specific amounts of these ingredients. If, for instance, the recipe calls for 6 eggs and you use 2, you are not going to achieve the desired result. If you leave out the sugar, you definitely won't achieve the desired result. That is why no matter how minor something may seem, it is still an important variable in the fitness recipe. I hope that helps explain the importance of executing all these directions exactly as specified.

If you do 4 days a week of resistance training but only 1 day every other week of cardiovascular training you will not achieve your goal. If you follow your diet to perfection but neglect the proper water intake you will not succeed. Remember, that by doing this, it may not happen overnight, but it will be the smartest, most effective, and most permanent way to become fit and lose fat.

Why lose over and over and over with gimmicky fads when you can do it right the first time and forget about it? It will become <u>habit</u> before you know it! Your body and mind will <u>crave</u> the healthy lifestyle and nothing else will do!

JUST SO YOU KNOW, GET READY TO BE THE BAD GUY

The funny thing about our society is that it reinforces an unhealthy lifestyle by saying, "its alright to indulge yourself." And those that are disciplined and serious about their fitness are made fun of and called compulsive fitness "freaks!" The paradox is that we glorify the look we achieve by taking our fitness seriously and treat those that do indulge as lazy or undisciplined social outcasts.

There will be times during your transformation that you will not be able to take part in activities, such as over-eating, when your family or friends are taking part in it. I remember one instance when my grandmother invited me over for dinner. This is a woman that was born in Naples, Italy and seems to always be cooking for 25 people or more. I walked in the door and the first thing she said was, "I am so glad to see you, I made your favorite lasagna!" Guess what? I couldn't eat lasagna that day. I said. "Nina (that's what I call her), I am on a special diet and cannot eat lasagna."

Of course, she thought I was crazy for being on a diet and said that I was already too skinny and insisted that I have some. When I pleaded with her to not tempt me and told her it would be alright if I had her chicken and salad, she saw that I was serious and honored my request. I can tell you one thing though, she was not happy but she got over it.

I had had my first taste of many more to come of being the bad guy. You will be in situations where you will be tempted by peers to eat and drink things that are not part of your new lifestyle. They will tease you at first…until they see your results, then they will envy you. The great thing is that once you become fit, you will be able to "cheat" periodically without the guilt or the consequences. So just prepare to be the bad guy.

Once your friends and family start to see how this lifestyle improves your life, they will understand. This is one of the reasons you should tell everyone beforehand what you are doing. Explain this to them and when you are at the end of your first journey, those same people that made fun, may just join you. Be a leader, dare to be different, dare to help others change for the better. And remember, one chicken wing won't kill you, but it's a start.

10 THINGS YOU MUST DO BEFORE YOU GET STARTED

1) LOOK AT YOURSELF IN THE MIRROR

One thing common with almost all humans is that when something about us does not make us happy, we try to block it out all together. One of the defining moments in my decision to change came when I saw pictures of myself in a bathing suit. Before this, I had no idea how bad I really looked. The day before you begin, don't laugh, take off all your clothes down to your undergarments and look at yourself in the mirror. And I am not saying just glance and cover up again, I mean LOOK AT YOURSELF.

Take about 5 minutes and look at every inch. Think to yourself "is this is really me?" Think about unleashing the person that is under there. Think about your visualization exercise and what you could be looking at. Think about how much better clothes will fit, think about how much more people will notice you, and think about how much better life is when you look good, think about how great it will feel to be FIT!

2) TELL PEOPLE WHAT YOU ARE DOING

I have mentioned this before as an important key to success. There are several reasons this is so. First of all, it helps with the "being the bad guy" thing, if people know what you are doing, they will prepare for it. Also, if you have to explain it every time a situation arises it can get pretty frustrating. If you tell everyone you are going to become fit and for some reason you try to rationalize why you should quit during your journey, you are going to look like an ass. Put some pressure on yourself. Initially you are going to need all the support you can get, so make sure your loved-ones know you need their support. Use them to get through the tough times.

The final reason for telling people that are close to you, is to hopefully find a partner. A partner is great for accountability purposes. Changing your life is much easier if your friend or spouse is taking the challenge with you!

3) WRITE YOURSELF A LETTER

Another effective trick to staying on track and supporting the realization part of the program is to write yourself a letter. This letter should be a totally honest list of why you <u>need</u> and want to change your life now. Be sure when writing this letter you are hard on yourself and do not sugar-coat anything. A few examples of what I wrote to myself in my letter are: "I have always wanted to see my abs; this is my shot to do it. If I don't start making positive changes now, I will be sorry when I get older. I will feel so much better if I am happy with the way I look. I want to spend quality time with my grandchildren when I am older. I don't want to be fat. I don't want to die of heart disease and I don't want diabetes. If I don't take action now it will be harder later."

I am sure you can come up with your own reasons. Don't be afraid to be brutally honest with yourself. This letter can then be put in a private place. No one ever needs to see it but you. When you feel like you want to give up, pull out the letter and reflect on it. It is powerful stuff! I guarantee it!

4) PICK A DAY TO BEGIN

Any journey needs a starting point. Starting is the hardest part of this entire program. Once you begin, make yourself a promise that no matter what the world throws at you, or what temptation you face, you will not quit. Tell yourself "I will overcome anything and never waiver. I am making a commitment that from this day forward I am going to strive for greatness in everything I do!"

Once you have all your planning and organization complete, and have entered the right state of mind, pick a day to start. I think Monday is the best day. That way you can have a last supper on Sunday and punish your body in anyway you want. Be sure that when you begin, you never quit.

I can't stand it when I tell people to just quit the bad habits and start the good ones. They always tell me it is not that simple! But that is the only simple way to do it! Cutting down on negative habits or using emotional crutches or hypnotists or therapists or whatever is complicated.

Making a mental commitment to yourself to just stop negative habits and start positive ones is the only simple way to do it. Every other way is complicated. Only you can do it!

5) BINGE ON YOUR FAVORITES

A couple days before you begin, go to the store or your favorite restaurant and binge on all of your favorites. Eat and drink to your heart's content. There are a couple reasons you do this and you can probably figure them out. If you eat and drink enough, it will be a long time before you want that crap again. Also, the carbohydrate loading will give you tons of energy for the next few days, minimizing the effects of dramatic change in diet. If you can get through the first few days with this program you are home-free.

The great thing about a healthy nutritional plan is that you will eat more often, with foods and drinks that are filling. The best thing about this program is you can binge once a week without any guilt or adverse effect. We call this the "Cheat Day or Free Day." I cover the Cheat Day in a later chapter.

6) YOU NEED A FITNESS JOURNAL

This goes back to the fail to prepare idea. A fitness journal is the history and log of your journey. Your journal should be with you everywhere you go. Everything you eat, everything you do, and every relevant emotion you feel should be written down in your journal. Motivational statements you hear can be written on the pages to keep you going when times get tough. Write down the time you wake up and the time you go to bed. Record the way you feel each day. If you feel tired, write it down, if you feel energetic, write it down. Be specific with your nutrition log. Don't just write down fish if you had fried fish. If you had salad dressing, record what kind. Record what time you ate and lifted or ran. Record all of your work-outs right down to the way they made you feel.

The logic behind this is if you record everything and you are lagging in certain aspects of your training and new lifestyle, you can refer back to your journal and investigate the problem. If you are not losing fat quickly enough and you look back at your journal entries and notice that you have not improved on your intensity levels during cardio work-outs you have your problem and can address it. If you are tired and you look back and see that you have been going to bed at 2 am and getting up at 6 a.m. you know you need to focus on your rest. The main three reasons you keep a journal are:

1   If you don't, you will be sorry you don't have a record of your journey when you have reached your goal.

2   It is much harder to eat BBQ chicken wings if you have to write them down in your journal.

3 It is hard to miss workouts when you have a space to fill.

7) TAKE ALL YOUR MEASUREMENTS

This is pretty much self-explanatory. Have someone take <u>all</u> your measurements. Only by recording your starting point can you efficiently strive to your goal. You should take new measurements every 4 weeks. This is a much better way to measure your improvement than weighing yourself. You will see, if you follow this program closely that the fat melts away pretty quickly and the lean muscle will begin to appear. After you weigh yourself on the day you begin, PUT YOUR SCALE IN THE CLOSET!

The main reason people fail at "dieting" is they rely so heavily on the scale. Muscle weighs a great deal more than fat so you can actually gain a little weight initially as you begin to get fitter. I cannot stress the importance of focusing on your fitness rather than your body weight. We have been wrongly conditioned for so many years to use weight as the proper measurement of health. WRONG!

The reduction of body fat and the improvement of lean muscle mass and cardiovascular strengthening is the true way to judge your fitness level. I will explain this in my next topic. Be sure to take accurate measurements of the following: Neck, Chest (relaxed and expanded), waist, hips, biceps (relaxed and flexed), forearms, thighs, and calves.

8) GET YOUR BODY FAT TESTED

As I mentioned in the previous section, your weight is not the best measurement of improvement. We quit most diets because after a couple weeks of dramatic weight loss we hit a wall and sometimes actually gain weight, this can be quite frustrating and usually leads to binge eating. The best measurement is a body fat test. There are several ways to do this; some are more accurate than others. The most common method is a skin-fold test. This test should be performed by a qualified professional. Skin is pinched and measured at several points over the body with a skin-fold caliper. Measurements can be taken on the back of the arm, upper back, waist, upper thigh, etc. These numbers are added together and put into a formula to reveal your body fat. This method is easy to obtain, but can be inaccurate by up to 5% more or less, and if done by someone that doesn't know what they are doing, results can be greatly skewed.

Another way is performed with a machine that measures your body fat by sending faint electrical charges through your body measuring your lean body mass. You input your weight, height and age, hold onto a couple sensors for a few seconds and *voila!* There's your body fat. The problem with this method is it can also be inaccurate from 3-5% and variables such as body heat, water retention and inaccuracy in weight and height, can dramatically affect your reading. Also these units can be very expensive.

The best way to measure your body fat is through hydrostatic weighing. This can be done at your local university, and some wellness centers may have one. For anywhere from $30-$75 you can get an exact measurement of your body composition. It is actually pretty simple. The test involves being suspended in a chair attached to a scale. Body density is calculated from the relationship of normal body weight to under water weight. Body fat percentage is calculated from body density. I suggest you cough up the cash and do this. I have met with clients that told me they just had their body fat tested at 15%

when in reality they were over 30%! They just went from "elite" to "obese!"

Here is a good explanation of why you should get your body fat tested and "focus on your fitness." You can lose a great deal of weight and actually become less fit. All crash dieting does is create a skinny, unfit person. It bothers me when I hear a thin person say they can eat anything they want and they never get fat. Let me tell you something, they may be thin on the outside, but they're not on the inside. A thin person can clog their arteries with fat just as an "overfat" person can.

Since I have implemented a healthy lifestyle, just about every weight chart I have looked at says I am overweight and in one case obese! Though I currently have a body fat level below 10% at 5'9" and 180 lbs! This puts me in the elite category of fitness level, but doctors who just follow a chart would tell me I had to lose weight!

Get on the scale at 45 and 90 days. After that I doubt you will get on a scale again. You can tell where you are just by looking in the mirror!

9) WRITE DOWN SPECIFIC GOALS

Again, if you fail to prepare, you should prepare to fail. You must write down at least 3 specific goals. I have explained in the Organize section the importance of this. Make these goals almost unattainable.

Some examples would be:

- Lower my body fat 10% in 90 days. This is a very attainable goal though initially it may seem miles away.
- Reduce my waist-line 4 inches in 90 days.
- Perform 50 push-ups /50 sit-ups

After you have written down these goals, write down the short term goals you must attain to achieve your long term ones.

In order to lower my body fat I must:

- Do 4 cardiovascular sessions per week.
- Eat 5-6 healthy meals per day.
- Do resistance training 4 days per week.

Put all these in your journal, so you can refer to them often while staying on track. It is important to remind yourself of why you are doing this. It is very easy to slack once you have begun to show dramatic improvement.

10) TAKE BEFORE PICTURES

This is the one everybody dreads. I cannot stress the importance of this simple task. Have a loved one, friend, or fitness professional take these pictures for you. The best choice of clothing is beach wear. Women can wear a sports bra and shorts. Men can also wear shorts. Take a picture from the front, side and back. If you want to pose, that is fine too but be sure to take good close-up pictures of the entire body. Remember, the worse they look the better. You will use these pictures not only for motivation, but when you are at the end of your journey, whether it be 90 days or 900 days, you will be so glad you have them. When you reach your 3 month to 1 year goal you will take the "after" pictures. As you have seen, there is nothing more powerful than a side by side comparison of a dramatic transformation.

WARNING: DO NOT EVEN ATTEMPT TO FOLLOW MY PROGRAM IF YOU HAVE A PROBLEM WITH TAKING A BEFORE PICTURE.

You are setting yourself up for failure and you are wasting your time.

THE "SECRET" FORMULAS

> Variety + Consistency + Discipline= Success
>
> Resistance Training + Aerobic Conditioning + Flexibility Training + Proper Nutrition + Water Intake + Rest + Positive Attitude = Total Fitness

If any of these components are neglected the end result will not be consistent. Think about it as a chemical formula. If any of the variables are lacking, you will not achieve optimal results. Why spend time in the gym to just feel better, when with the same amount of output you can achieve greatness. People fail to realize that by following the old myths of fitness they are actually working too hard and achieving less. When by avoiding common problems they can actual eat more and work-out less to achieve maximum results.

I can remember towards the end of my transformation someone at the gym asked me how I achieved such amazing results so quickly. He followed his question immediately with this statement: "I have followed the same routine for 5 years, 5 days a week, 2 hours a day, and I have yet to see improvement."

I began to explain how he had wasted his time if he was looking for improvement. I tried to explain to him how the body adapts to whatever it is doing and how it needs to be shocked periodically to overcome plateaus. Before I could finish telling him about short, intense sessions with less socializing and more exercising, he became defensive and explained how he lifted just to feel better. I told him I thought that was great, but why not improve <u>and</u> feel better by doing less in less time?

I see the same mistakes with diet. People starve themselves or eat things that they don't like or eat things they think are healthy that really aren't when they could eat tasty foods and more calories if they just did a little research.

MYTHS DISPELLED! EXCUSES ADDRESSED!

"IF I DO A LOT OF ABDOMINAL EXERCISES I WILL GET GREAT ABS!"

This is somewhat true, but all the ab-machine companies have distorted this…almost everyone has pretty good abs already, in order to walk upright, your abdominal muscles are always working. It is true that doing ab-work will define and build your abdominal muscles, but if you don't watch what you eat and perform high intensity cardiovascular exercises, fat will always cover your great abs.

"WOMEN SHOULDN'T WEIGHT TRAIN BECAUSE THEY WILL BUILD BIG BULKY MUSCLES"

This is one of the biggest misconceptions of exercise. It is just as important for women to perform resistance exercises to maintain their overall health as men. Building lean muscle can make the female body look more shapely not to mention the jolt new muscle gives to the metabolism. Plus for every pound of muscle you build, you burn an extra 50 calories. Unless a women is performing heavy sets of power type exercises like the squat, dead lift and bench press and eating like a pig they will never build a masculine physique.

"IF I DO A LOT OF SETS OF HIGH REPETITION EXERCISES I WILL TONE."

First of all, I don't know what this means to work-out for tone. The trick is to change your work-out up often to create muscle confusion. Some work-outs should be fewer repetitions with more weight while other work-outs can be quick intense sessions with high reps. High reps and lower weights will develop muscle endurance, low reps and higher weights develop muscular strength. Seeing the muscle or being "toned" is a matter of any weight training and proper diet. I have lifted heavy for a long period and cut my calorie intake and developed quite a lean and strong physique.

"IF I DON'T EAT THAT MUCH I WILL LOSE WEIGHT."

While over a long-period of time this may be true, it is not the most effective way to lose fat and get fit. As I will mention in the next section, it is imperative to keep the body-furnace going along with weight training and cardiovascular training to optimize fat-loss. If I cut my calories I will lose weight initially, but I will continue to store fat. Your body actually thinks it is starving. If you eat many small meals throughout the day, your body will adapt by knowing you have a constant supply of nutrition. This will allow your body to burn stored fat because it knows you will be getting more food in a short time. And by doing resistance work, your body will burn fat instead of muscle for energy.

"LONG DISTANCE RUNNING IS THE BEST WAY TO GET INTO SHAPE."

The runners are going to hate me, but I don't see many positive reasons to run long-distances. The only reason for running long-distances is the feeling you get from your endorphin rush. Many runners talk about how they get a high from running. They also get knee and foot problems and running is not the best for developing a powerful and attractive physique. Look at the body of a World-Class marathon runner. They tend to have little muscle definition and be quite slight in appearance. Now look at a World-Class Sprinter, they are incredibly muscular, have low body-fat and appear to be very powerful. In a later chapter I will explain the benefits of High Intensity Interval Training (HIIT). Unless you have the urge to run a marathon or 10K, there is no health need to run long distances at a

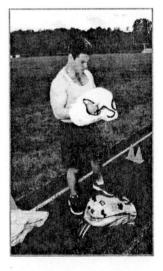

Training at your local high school can bring back your youthful mind set.

constant pace. Hop on your bike for a ride in the country or go out to your local high school and run the bleachers if you want to get fit.

"LOTS OF PASTA IS GOOD FOR YOU."
Wrong. Enough said.

"LIFTING WEIGHTS EVERYDAY WILL GET ME MY RESULTS MUCH MORE QUICKLY"

I have seen people in the gym training like crazy for years and never improve. They lift everyday, they lift hard and they never get anywhere! Rest is just as important as training. Your muscles and body need to rest in order to grow. You should never exercise the same muscle group in consecutive days. This will lead to over-training, where you can develop cold-like symptoms, and exercise related injuries. If you do the same type of cardiovascular training all the time, switch it up every 4 or 5 days.

"NO-CARB, HIGH PROTEIN DIETS ARE THE MOST EFFECTIVE WAY TO LOSE WEIGHT."

Stay away from them. I won't go into much detail about the nasty effect this type of eating can have on your body, not to mention how gross it is to just eat meat, cheese and eggs. What I will tell you is that carbohydrates are a necessary part of anyone's diet. Once you have cut your carbs, your body goes into a state of Ketosis. Your body only has a couple of places to get energy. Carbs are the quickest and fat is the next choice, unless you are not working out, and then it takes a little from your muscle each day. After your body adjusts to just protein and no carbs your body becomes carbohydrate sensitive. So when you have lost your initial 15 or 20 pounds (most of which will be fluids) and you begin to eat properly again you will inevitably gain back your weight plus more. Your body will crave carbs so much because you have deprived yourself of them, that that is all you will want to eat. I admit that in order to quickly lose that last few pounds of body fat, a low-carb high protein diet is perfect. Following this diet any longer than 7-14 days can lead to disaster.

"I NEED TO SPEND A COUPLE HOURS IN THE GYM TO GET RESULTS."

This is totally crazy. The biggest mistake most people make in the gym is they spend too much time there. Get in and get out! Wear headphones so people are not likely to speak to you. Go from one exercise to the next with short breaks in between. Have a game plan by knowing exactly what you are going to do once you get there. Don't waste time with idle chit-chat. If you are taking longer than 60 minutes for your work-out, and this includes warm-up, stretching, weight training, cool-down and cardiovascular training, your either doing too many exercises, taking too much of a break, or socializing too much.

"I NEED TO LOSE WEIGHT BEFORE I START EXERCISING"

I can't even believe I am entertaining this myth but I have heard it so much lately I guess there is a need. By just trying to lose fat through dieting you are missing the boat. The time to start exercising is NOW. By exercising on a regular basis you will not only lose fat at a much higher rate, but it is easier to follow a nutritional plan if you are working out. And always remember, exercise is a self-competitive activity. You should never look at someone else as the norm. If you feel self-conscious about your weight...get over it! Who cares what people think, show people you have the courage to lead your own life on your terms. If you still have an issue, work-out at home.

"ONCE I QUIT SMOKING / KIDS ARE OLDER/ BUSINESS GET GOING / JOIN A GYM / I WILL BEGIN AN EXERCISE PROGRAM."

Excuses, excuses, excuses! You need to take action now.

"I AM TOO FAR OUT OF SHAPE TO START NOW."

Stop it! You can always do something. If you are dramatically over-weight and out of shape, start slowly. Do a few light exercises a day and begin by cutting out one bad thing, like soda, or fast food, or eating late and you will see that before you know it you are able to begin a rigorous program. Our bodies are very forgiving. You can be way out of control and less than a year later you can be training your butt off, literally!

There is a great riddle to illustrate this:

Question: How does a mouse eat an elephant?
Answer: One bite at a time.

DON'T MAKE EXCUSES and DON'T FALL FOR THE MYTHS!

CHAPTER 5

NUTRITION: WHAT AND HOW TO EAT

What you eat has so many effects on how you live your life. It is amazing that we are not more selective. A proper nutritional plan can not only reduce the waist-line but make other dramatic improvements in our lifestyle that we seldom think about. By eating a healthy diet we can increase our productivity, enhance our mood and reduce the effects of depression. I don't think I have to go into how a healthy diet reduces the chances of long-term illness that can have some nasty effects on our bodies as we get older. Things like diabetes, cardiovascular disease and cancers can all be blamed, for the most part on an abusive diet and lack of movement.

Eating great can be a very rewarding experience if we just train our bodies to adapt to the proper foods. Our bodies will crave whatever we are eating. If we are eating fat, salt and sugar, that is what our bodies will crave. If we eat fruits, vegetables, lean meats and fish, that is what our bodies will crave. We must realize that eating is not something to do when you are bored or depressed. It is <u>fuel</u> that we need to exist at the highest level possible. Don't get me wrong, it is alright to treat yourself to a cheeseburger and fries every so often, but to make it the staple of your diet can have catastrophic effects on the way our bodies function.

The frequency of our meals and size can have just as dramatic effect on our body as the amount of calories we are consuming. Since our physiologies are designed to be efficient hunters and gatherers we get optimal nutritional intake by eating smaller meals more often throughout the day.

There are several physiological and psychological advantages to doing this. First, by eating smaller meals more often, our bodies continue to burn fuel because it is trained to know there will be another meal just a couple hours down the road. This speeds up our metabolism and leads to more efficient fat burning. Also by eating more often our energy level is elevated to keep up with our metabolism. By eating smaller meals we avoid that full, lethargic feeling we get when we eat too much and too many bad carbohydrates. The "American" style of eating big meals late in the day leads to what is called a lazy metabolism. Psychologically, eating smaller meals more often works best because there is such a short time between meals. Even if we begin to feel hungry we can be assured that we can eat again in an hour or so.

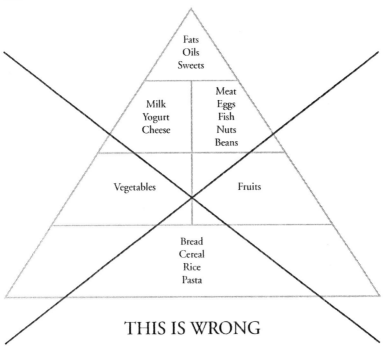

Fats
Oils
Sweets

Milk
Yogurt
Cheese

Meat
Eggs
Fish
Nuts
Beans

Vegetables

Fruits

Bread
Cereal
Rice
Pasta

THIS IS WRONG

THE FDA FOOD PYRAMID IS WRONG!

I don't even want to spend any time going into the problems with how the FDA suggests we eat. I don't know who came up with this idea, but it almost seems it was designed to make people fat. Anyone who is eating 12 servings of breads, cereals or pasta a day while living a sedentary lifestyle will show you that this is not the right way to eat.

By eating starchy, high-carbohydrate foods (especially those that contain refined sugars), we are setting ourselves up for disaster. These types of foods create high spikes in blood sugar. The body reacts with a surge of insulin into your system. That insulin forces glucose from your blood and into your muscle and fat cells. Your blood sugar levels then drop and before you know it you feel hungry again.

On the other hand, whole-grain foods have a slower more steady effect on blood sugar and your insulin levels, these types of foods make you feel full, longer. I could have an entire chapter on the problems with the food pyramid and all the myths associated with proper nutrition, but I will save you the boredom. Instead, I will outline and illustrate the correct balance of nutritional intake as dictated by our body chemistry.

We know that exercise is the foundation of any wellness program. By exercising regularly you will see that your body will crave more densely nutritious foods. The best thing is that when you do cheat, there will be little effect because of the speed of your metabolism. Plus your body will be trained to know that it is going to receive more nutrition so it will pass the junk through your body more quickly.

The Food Pyramid below is the one that works.

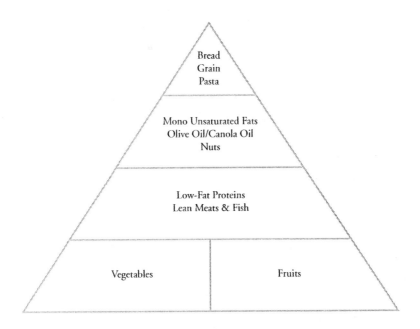

Bread
Grain
Pasta

Mono Unsaturated Fats
Olive Oil/Canola Oil
Nuts

Low-Fat Proteins
Lean Meats & Fish

Vegetables

Fruits

THE RIGHT FOOD PYRAMID

The bottom line is this: If your goal is to just lose fat this is as simple as it gets. I would suggest to someone that is working out regularly and properly that they should eat between 1800 and 2400 calories per day. If you are a male training really hard you can get away with more. But the simplicity of it is this: if you are burning 3000 calories per day, and eating 3500 calories a day, you will gain 1 pound of fat per week. On the other hand, if you are eating 2500 calories per day and burning 3000 you will lose one pound of fat per week. Rocket science huh?

IN MORE DETAIL

Water	*Drink plenty of water!*

Fish/Seafood/Poultry/Eggs	*2-3 servings/day*

Dairy	*1-2 servings/day*
(Milk is a food, not a drink!)	

Nuts, Legumes	*2-3 servings/day*
(Almonds, Black Beans, Chick Peas, Red Beans)	

Fruit and Veggies	*3-5 servings each daily*
(No potatoes, no corn, no carrots.	
Eat broccoli, eggplant, cauliflower, romaine lettuce, etc.)	

Fat	*In moderation*
(Olive oil, and most poly or mono unsaturated oils)	

Whole Grains	*A little with each meal*
(Brown rice, oatmeal, wheat bread, cous cous)	

People say that they don't know what to eat or how to eat healthy, that is a bunch of you know what! They just don't want to learn. Here is another excuse I have heard why people don't eat properly:

"I can't afford to eat nutritiously."

Hogwash! You can't afford <u>not</u> to eat nutritiously.

I saw a special on TV recently about overweight children and their distressed mothers. The mothers will complain that their doctors had warned them that their children had a weight problem and needed to change their diet. When these mothers journeyed to the store they were shocked at the cost of healthy foods compared to less nutritious processed foods. She continued to buy the junk while insisting the nutritious food was not in her family's budget.

Her main comparison was white bread vs. whole grain bread. She argued that a loaf of white bread was around 99 cents and the whole grain was $2.39! I find that by investigating a little further the face value is rarely true. While her 12 year old, 265 pound son looked on, she admitted that that loaf of white bread would rarely make it through the day!

I guarantee the whole grain will last much longer; not to mention the whole grain bread's nutritional superiority. The truth was they really couldn't afford the junk. The reason: they were eating 5 times the amount of food they needed! If we don't set a healthy example for our children, we are abusing them. And I am not even going to go into the amount that obesity related health problems cost the health care system annually!

Overall, boxed meals, family dinners and fast food may seem more of a value but this is far from true. Over the course of a month, the junk food menu will cost an average of 4 times more than the healthy menu. The same person that can eat a whole

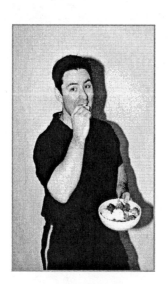

Broccoli and Cauliflower are great ways to fill up!

loaf of white bread or an entire bag of chips will find it difficult to polish off a whole bag of whole grain bread or cauliflower! When people say to me that they never feel full I tell them it is because of your food choices. Grab a pound of broccoli and eat to your heart's content. You'll feel full before you know it.

Your body naturally craves foods high in fat, salt and sugar, so it may seem more satisfying initially than a healthy meal. As I have said before, eating high fat or starchy food tastes good but the full feeling is short lived, followed by renewed hunger. In turn, when your body is getting the proper amount of nutrition through fiber, lean meat and green veggies you are doing two positive things. Not only are you getting 10 times the nutritional value with fewer calories, you will become satisfied more quickly and remain full longer. EAT FOR FUEL not PLEASURE!

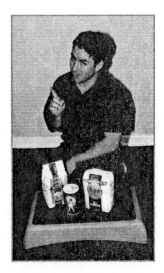

The Three No's: Sugar, Salt, and Flour

You will be amazed that once you have implemented this healthy lifestyle you will be more creative with food selection and preparation. You may even be surprised at how great a healthy meal can taste! You have to admit that cheeseburgers, pizza, french fries, sweets and soda all sound like a great idea at the time, but feeling full, bloated and guilty is the punishment for your short-lived enjoyment.

You will never miss that sleepy, bloated feeling you get immediately after eating junk. There is one thing for sure, not only will you feel so much better after eating a healthy meal, but it is all guilt free!

PAY ATTENTION TO SERVING SIZE<u>!</u>

Many people think that a serving is what you are served! The truth is that most restaurants give you 3-4 times as much food as you should be eating at one sitting. During the day, most people consume way too many servings of pasta, bread, potatoes, and red meats and too few servings of fish, fruits and green vegetables.

A popular sandwich franchise markets itself as a healthy choice for lunch. Though this may be true for a couple of their choices, most people eat a large sandwich with mayonnaise a side of chips and a sugary iced tea or fruit drink. This multiple serving combination can pack a big punch when it comes to calories and sugar. I am not saying that you can't eat out and eat healthy; you can. I just want you to be aware of what the average person is doing and how you can sabotage your healthy diet. There are many hidden items that through the years have been looked at as healthy alternatives but are really bad. Baked chips may sound like a healthy choice to the deep fried version, but the truth is that <u>both</u> are terrible and should be avoided at all costs. Also, be careful with sport drinks and sweetened teas. They can be just as bad as soft drinks.

THE TRUE MEASURE OF A "SERVING"

Meat, Poultry, Fish, Beans and Eggs

2-3 oz. of cooked lean meat, poultry or fish

1 cup of cooked beans

1 egg

Bread, Cereal, Rice and Pasta

1 slice of bread

1 cup of cooked rice or pasta

1 oz. cold cereal

Milk, Yogurt, Cheese

1 cup of milk

1.5 oz. of natural cheese

Vegetables

1 cup of leafy vegetables

1 cup other veggies, cooked

Fruit

1 medium apple or orange

1 cupped handful of grapes

DEFINITELY EAT THESE	*DON'T EAT THESE*
Lean meats and fish	Fried foods
Green veggies	Refined grain products
Fruit	Butter and margarine
Low-fat dairy	Whole milk
Legumes	Carbonated beverages
Wheat wraps	Fruit juice
Wheat pasta	Sugar
Egg whites	Alcohol
	Salty foods

INSTEAD OF THESE...	*EAT THESE*
White rice	Brown rice
White bread	Whole-grain bread
Pasta	Whole-grain pasta
Steak	Fish
Potatoes	Legumes
Chips	Pretzels
Cookies	Graham crackers
Ground Beef	Ground Turkey
Whole Milk	Skim Milk
Eggs	Egg substitute (Eggs Beaters)
Kool Aid	Crystal Lite
Crisco	Olive Oil

We still think that eating 6-12 servings of bread and pasta is good for us. When I advise someone to cut down on the pasta I always hear the same thing. "Pasta is good for you." "It's fat free." When I say that a serving or two of pasta is alright but too much leads to fat they immediately disagree. Most people think a trip to the local Italian restaurant franchise is a healthy choice. In reality, the average pasta portion is about 4 servings in one sitting! That's not even including the bread sticks and meat or cream sauce that covers your pasta!

People will drink glass after glass of juice or eat fruit yogurt or fat free snacks and think they are dieting. Most juices and yogurts are loaded with sugar, avoid them at all costs. Fat-free high carbohydrate snacks are horrible for you. Not only can you eat them until they are gone, because there is nothing to make you feel full, but they are loaded with sugar and nasty things to make them taste good. Just because something does not have fat in it does not mean it won't make you fat.

THE GROCERY LIST

HAVE THESE IN THE HOUSE AND NOTHING ELSE!

*Always eat before you go to the grocery store!

Vegetables	Fruits	Carbs	Proteins	Fats	Condiments
Artichoke	Apricots	All-Bran	Chicken Breasts	Almonds	Mustard
Asparagus	Blue Berries	Brown Rice	Cod	Canola Oil	Salsa
Broccoli	Cantaloupe	Couscous	Cottage Cheese	Olives	Vinegar/ Olive Oil
Brussels Sprouts	Cranberries	Legumes/ Beans	Egg Beaters	Olive Oil	
Cauliflower	Granny Smith Apples	Lentils	Flank Steak	PAM	
Celery	Grapes	Oatmeal	Flounder		
Lettuce (Iceberg)	Grapefruit	Spinach Noodles	Lobster		
Lettuce (Romaine)	Honeydew Melon	Total Cereal	Low-Fat Plain Yogurt		
Mushrooms	Kiwi	Wheat Pasta	Roughy		
Onion	Lemons	Wheat Wraps	Salmon		
Peppers	Orange		Scallops		
Eggplant			Sea Bass		
Spinach			Skim Milk		
Tomato			Snapper		
Yams			Sole		
Zucchini			Trout		
			Tuna		
			Turkey Breasts		

NOTHING TASTES AS GOOD AS IT FEELS TO BE FIT

GET RID OF TEMPTATION!

Once you have learned which foods are good for you and which are bad it's time to clean out the cupboards. Take all the junk and give it away or throw it out. Take temptation out of the equation and you have already won half the battle. You are much more likely to crave something if you have it.

People with children argue with me that they have the cookies and chips "for the kids." Well first of all, your kids don't need that crap either. We develop our fitness habits at a very young age. If we teach our kids to eat junk that is what they will want as they develop into adults. Fruits are just as tasty if not tastier than cookies or snack cakes. Your kids may argue at first, but they will thank you later.

If your spouse isn't on the same page as you...yet, give him his own cupboard...and don't go in it. Once he or she sees you changing for the better he or she will soon join you, I guarantee it. I know I said you don't need any nutrition products to accomplish your transformation, and you don't, but meal replacement nutritional bars can make your daily eating much easier. I throw a couple bars in my glove-box or in my gym bag to eat for my in-between meals. The problem with eating "food" six to eight times a day is it can get tough to eat that much!

There are many companies out there that produce delicious and healthy nutrition bars or drinks. If you are trying to drop body fat and just build a little muscle I suggest the nutritional line of Zone Bars, they taste very good and have a perfect mix of protein, carbs and fat.

If you are training hard and wish to put on some muscle, I like the Myoplex Deluxe Peanut Butter and Chocolate bar from EAS. These bars can really curb your craving for sweets while providing the proper nutrient mix you need to lose fat and build muscle. They are relatively inexpensive compared to the same amount of food and can go down easy after a tough work-out. I strongly suggest though, that you only use these bars as a snack and never a meal.

EAT REAL FOOD FOR YOUR MAIN MEALS! Buy a few different ones to see which tastes best to you. Stay away from bars with too many carbs and too much sugar. Unless you are a long-distance runner or hiker and need to maintain a high carbohydrate diet, don't eat meal replacement shakes or bars with over 25 grams of carbs and 300 calories. Powerbars and Cliff Bars are like candy bars in your body, they are great when you need a lot of calories and carbohydrates in a small package, but they don't make the best snack.

ORGANIZE YOUR MEAL PLAN. This is easier than it sounds. I will include some recipes for you to use later in the book, but as long as you are adhering to the food suggestions you can use just about any combination without making a mistake. Just be sure to eat a carb, protein and veggie with every meal. Remember you are working to ultimately eat 6 meals per day. Here is how you do it:

Meal 1 (8 a.m.)	Breakfast, 500 calories (oatmeal, 2 egg beaters with spinach or half a grapefruit
Meal 2 (10 a.m.)	Snack, 250 calories (nutrition bar)
Meal 3 (1 p.m.)	Meal, 300 calories (Chicken Wrap w/spinach, side of brown rice and a granny smith apple)
Meal 4 (3 p.m.)	Snack, 250 calories (Cottage Cheese/ Yogurt w/berries, bar)
Meal 5 (6 p.m.)	Dinner, 400 calories (Fish Jambalaya w/ Red Beans, rice, Eggplant, and Tomatoes)
Meal 6 (8-9 p.m.)	High Protein Snack, 250 calories (Whey Protein Drink with skim milk, a few slices of Turkey and half a cup of cottage cheese make a great evening snack. I prefer a basic protein drink available at any nutrition retail store.)

It is easier than you think and under 2000 calories without ever being hungry! You can throw any combination of lean meat, beans and veggies in a wheat wrap and you're ready to go! Throw a little salsa in there and you have a tasty, quick and healthy meal. Remember, <u>you are eating for fuel</u>. Once you develop this mentality you will feel like a million bucks. You will sleep better, have more energy, and be in a more even and positive mood. Once you get the hang of things and begin to see and feel change, eating well will become easier and easier. I see many of my clients actually becoming more conscious than me when it comes to reading labels and being alert to food.

Food is a drug and when abused can be deadly. It amazes me that people eat things that contain ingredients that they have no idea what they are. If you are training hard, here is a great food plan for optimal nutritional intake that will lead to optimal fitness performance:

Meal 1: High Protein/ moderate complex carb/ low fat

Meal 2: Moderate Protein/ low carb/ low fat

Meal 3: High Protein/ low carb/ moderate fat

Meal 4: (Pre-workout) High complex carb/ moderate
protein. This will raise your glycogen levels giving
you that extra needed energy for your workout.

Meal 5: (Post-workout) Replenish lost nutrients with 50
grams of simple and complex carbs with 50 grams
of protein.

Meal 6: High Protein/ low carb/ moderate fat

Late Snack: Whey Protein Shake (I like the strawberry
from EAS)

LOOK AT THE LABELS! Before you know it you will learn the exact nutrition break-downs of all your favorite healthy foods.

Remember the basic trick is to just be sure and eat a complex carb with a protein at every meal, except your late night snack which should be a protein. Try not to eat 3 hours before bed and you will see that the fat will disappear by just doing that and not changing anything else

YOUR PLATE SHOULD LOOK LIKE THIS

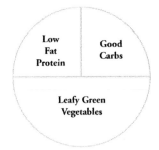

All meals should consist of equal parts lean proteins, good carbohydrates, and leafy green vegetables.

QUICK TIPS

- Don't drink anything while you eat
- Drink a glass of water 15 minutes before and immediately after a meal.
- Chew.
- Snack on cucumber, celery and apple slices.
- Pre-prepare your meals. (Use plastic storage containers to control your portions.)
- Keep healthy snacks with you
- Do something when commercials feature food!
- Stay busy.
- Take a Cheat Day
- Stay on the outside aisles of the grocery store.
- Watch out for hidden killers. (Soy sauce, ketchup, and sodium)

CHAPTER 6

EXERCISING: WHAT TO DO AND HOW TO DO IT

One thing that I have found about exercising is that pretty much whatever you do that incorporates resistance training and aerobic training will lead to improvement in health. The most important thing to realize for those of you that have found it difficult to stick to your training is that you should concentrate initially on what you enjoy doing.

Don't put together some crazy program that consists of exercises that you know are good for you but you hate! You'll never do them. It is better to start off simply with easy exercises that you enjoy and will set a strong foundation for improving to the next level. If you are currently totally sedentary, anything that you do to work your muscles and heart will be a marked improvement. Just moving a little more than normal can help dramatically improve the quality of your life.

Don't put so much stress on yourself in the beginning to succeed that you end up quitting. I have seen so many people begin with all the best intentions in the world only to quit because of over-training. Also, there is nothing worse than getting so excited about exercise that you hurt yourself or train so hard you have to take a week to recover. On the other hand, make sure your work-out session is intense enough that you raise your heart rate and push yourself a little.

One thing experts have been arguing about forever is what work-out works best for each individual. They have always said that there is no one work-out that works for everyone. Specifically they are right, but by taking a broader more philosophical look, there are two work-outs that will work for everyone no matter what you body-type, experience and goals are. The first one that works is the one you will do.

If you won't do it, you can have the best program in the world, and never succeed. What I have found works best for myself and most of my clients is this: Because I get bored easily and prefer a higher intensity level when exercising I implement great variety into my program design. It keeps me interested and is always shocking my muscles into improvement.

Variety, Consistency, and Intensity are Key!

As I have said before, our bodies are extremely adaptable. If you do the same thing over and over your body will begin to adapt, ending in frustrating plateaus. If you become too regimented in the type of activities you do, the number of repetitions, the weights, or exercise intensity, you will never improve. Not only is this method of exercise counterproductive in achieving new goals, it's also boring. Always have a game plan when it comes to daily exercise but be sure to change it up often. I will break down the three components to explain them further.

VARIETY

Everyone knows what variety is, but how does it apply to total fitness? People have thought forever that lifting heavy weights for fewer reps will produce bulky muscle growth and doing lighter weights and more repetitions will produce a more toned look. In some ways this is true but for the most part there are so many factors and variables that can affect target muscle building.

For instance, if I lift heavy all the time with just a few reps I will build bigger stronger muscles, but I may also set myself up for injury by over-training at this method. By lifting heavy and increasing my cardio and reducing calories I will achieve a "toned" look.

On the other hand, if I perform a toning specific weight program with lots of sets and reps, but I fail to do my cardio or I eat 5000 calories a day I doubt I will ever appear toned. This is why I preach variety. If I change my work-outs every couple weeks or once a month I will not only achieve results more quickly, I will lessen my chances of feeling bored and over-training.

Some weeks lift heavier weights, fewer reps with longer rests between sets. Some months lift lighter weights, with increased reps and shorter rests between sets. When you want to put on size, decrease your cardio work, increase your calorie intake and lift heavier. When you want to get lean, increase your cardio work and decrease your calorie intake. It is as simple as that! Always be sure to change up your exercises in order to recruit new muscle fiber. I will go into more detail about specific exercises later on in the chapter.

CONSISTENCY

I suggest a minimum of 3 good resistance work-outs per week to get anything noticeable out of them. 4-5 short sessions is actually optimal. If you are an experienced and fit athlete, you can get away with 2 VERY intense work-outs per week. Your resistance training work-outs should always consist of these four components:

1 Warm-up	10 minutes on a treadmill, exercise bike, or walking
2 Stretching	5-15 minutes of light, gentle, overall body stretching
3 Resistance Training	15-25 minutes of resistance exercises
4 Cool-Down	5-? minutes on a treadmill or bike at low rate

These four components should be present at each work-out whether they are at home or at the gym. Again, remember that by leaving out any variable, no matter how small it may seem to be, will aid in setting yourself up for failure and hinder you in achieving optimal results. Make your work-outs a priority in your life. Instead of trying to find time to workout, MAKE TIME! You will see that just by being consistent in your work-outs you will feel and look a million times better in a short time.

INTENSITY

Your level of intensity is directly related to your current fitness level. The trick is to exercise hard enough that you improve, but not so hard that you hurt yourself or pass out. The more you train, the more you will begin to get a feel for how hard you should be pushing yourself. It is difficult initially because you may always feel out of breath or weak, so your exercise intensity level will be difficult to monitor. I use this method to check my aerobic threshold. If I have difficulty carrying on a brief conversation with someone while training my cardio system I will ease off. I test my intensity with weight training in this fashion, if I have difficulty

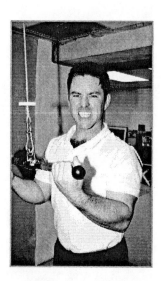

Intensity will help your get the most out of your workout.

catching my breath after 15 seconds of rest, or if I cannot perform another identical set after 90 seconds of rest, I have either exhausted that muscle or I need to turn it down a bit.

Also, be sure to stretch before, during and after exercise. This will help produce longer leaner looking muscles while reducing the pain or muscle burn associated with weight training. Stretching also is paramount in preventing injuries and insuring overall fitness. <u>Take stretching seriously</u>! It is vital to your health. Don't push it aside.

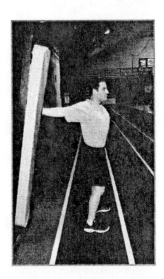

Don't forget to stretch!

On the following pages I am going to go into detail about the work-out. I strongly suggest that you stick as closely as possible to my exact program. It may seem very easy initially but it is incredibly effective. I have designed two different work-outs. One work-out is for those of you that have access to a health club or gym, and the other is for those of you who do not and must train at home.

Although it is not totally necessary to join a health club, I would advise you to find somewhere that is convenient and become a member. There are several reasons for this.

First, you will put yourself in a positive environment with other health conscious people. If you are self-conscious about working out with others, don't be! You are competing with yourself. If you think people will look at you funny, good, they might! Put on your headphones and go to work. Use them as motivation to reach your goal. You will want people to look at you soon enough.

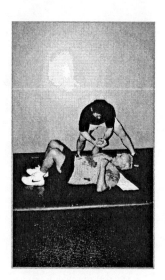

Working out with others offers fun and encouragement

Another reason to join a club or gym is that you will have some sort of supervision. Though I have found that most people don't know much about proper fitness, even in the clubs, there is a chance you will run into someone that knows their stuff and will be willing to help. At the least, you may find someone that can help you when you need it.

Another plus to working out at a facility is that you will have access to the right equipment. This adds to the variety of choices you will have so your workouts will remain interesting and ever-changing. Most clubs also offer some great classes like aerobics or Pilates that can aid in your overall transformation.

The most important reason to join a club is that it is somewhere you feel obligated to go because you are paying and there is little outside distraction. By training at home there is always a phone that could ring or a visitor that may stop over. For those of you that don't think it is in your budget, cancel your cable and focus on your priorities! There are many clubs out there that you can join for under a buck a day!

I have separated this program into 4 phases. Depending on your current fitness level you could spend 2 to 6 weeks of training in each phase. It is very important to educate yourself whenever possible on proper fitness. Read everything you can. This is important for a couple of reasons. First, it puts you in the proper state-of-mind to effectively change your lifestyle. If you are constantly reading about health and seeing healthy people you will begin to change the way you think.

Secondly, you will gain important knowledge of your most precious and valuable asset: <u>your health!</u> When you are done with your first 90 days you will find that you have become an expert when it comes to your body. You will know when to ease off, when to increase your intensity, what exercises give you the best results, and what time of day you train the best. You will also learn what your strengths and weaknesses are, therefore you can adjust accordingly. <u>Knowledge is power</u>!

It amazes me that the majority of people know more about how a computer works than how their body works, or how a plant should be taken care of when they have no idea of how to take care of themselves!

The greatest thing about exercise is that once you have put your time in and reached your goals it does not take much to maintain. You will have to do little more than walk a few minutes a day, and exercise 2 times a week in order to keep what you have. I have yet to see someone who became fit who didn't continue to set higher goals. It just gets easier and easier!

THE WORKOUT

In order to get optimal results I advise my clients to do their fat-burning cardio session when they wake-up on an empty stomach. The reason for this is you are burning stored calories rather than calories you have eaten throughout the day so you will burn more fat. I know it can be tough to train twice a day but it is not impossible. Also, by doing light aerobic training in the morning you will see that the rest of your day will be great!

It is also optimal to do your weight training in early afternoon. Again, I know this can be tough. We are talking about being optimal here. If you must do your work-outs at one time, do your resistance training first, followed by your cardio fitness. The reason for this is you can really use the energy you have stored to lift weights. By lifting weights first you will efficiently deplete your energy stores, leaving only fat to be burned during cardiovascular training.

Remember to adhere as closely to my program as possible for the first 90 days. Once you have transformed yourself, you will see that you can design programs on your own.

Before every work-out be sure to have a game plan and adhere to it as closely as possible.

THINGS TO REMEMBER WHEN WORKING OUT

1) REPETITIONS AND SETS

A repetition is the performance of one action of the exercise itself. A set is the total amount of repetitions for an exercise. For example 2 sets of 15 reps of bicep curls would be performing the exercise 15 times consecutively, then resting for the specified period, and then completing another 15 repetitions.

2) RESTING

When completing each exercise, you should rest for 1 minute between sets. Resting less won't give your body enough time to recover, and resting more won't maximize the benefit of the exercise. Between exercises you should rest for 2 minutes.

3) BREATHING

This may sound really obvious– but breathe! You'd be amazed how many people try to hold their breath while lifting or forget to think about their breathing while working out. A good way to think about it is to EXHALE WHILE EXERTING. For example, if you are doing chest press exercises, exhale as you push the weights away from your body, and inhale as you bring them back. This is true for all exercises.

4) HOW MUCH WEIGHT SHOULD YOU USE?

The proper weight is that which can be lifted the target amount of reps with the last rep being almost impossible to complete.

LET'S GO!

I am going to suggest four types of work-outs that will be very effective, two for training at home and two in the gym. The first is a full length workout consisting of four Phases. I will call this the Primary Workout. The second is an Abbreviated Workout that if done with the proper intensity will be plenty to get your butt in shape. Don't be fooled by the abbreviated training method. It doesn't take very long, but it hits all your muscle groups effectively.

HIIT

Before I walk through the workouts I need to familiarize you with the idea of HIIT which is included in several of the workout phases.

HIIT means High Intensity Interval Training. This is my favorite way to train and experts everywhere are praising the results from this type of training while stating that nagging injuries are few and far between. I will go into a specific explanation in Phase II.

Basically HIIT is designed to raise and lower the heart rate at specific intervals. As an example: walking up and down hills, or sprinting for a short burst then walking for a short period. This method is much more effective than long distance training for several reasons. Not only will HIIT increase your explosive power and burn body fat more efficiently, but your chances of getting a joint injury are virtually non-existent.

During Phase I you will not being doing HIIT. You instead will be training your muscles to get used to what you are going to be doing. This step is designed to develop muscle memory, proper form and condition your muscles for what lies ahead in future phases.

It is very important not to over do it too much during the first week or so of this phase. It may seem easy at first, but it is designed to prepare your body for the more intense latter phases. If by the second week you are not experiencing any severe muscle soreness, shortness of breath, or light headedness you can go on to Phase II. Phase I is also important for strengthening your heart and preparing it for your HIIT sessions.

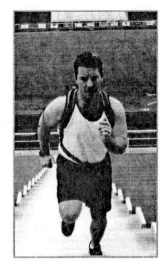

Running stairs is also an excellent HIIT method.

Outside of the physical aspects of HIIT, psychologically I believe it is more effective because it is not as boring as longer distance endurance training. You push yourself for a short time, then rest. You have several short term goals instead of one long-term goal. Instead of thinking about the 45 minutes ahead or the 5 miles still to go, all you have to focus on is a short distance or short time.

Long distance training can get boring, plus it isn't very good for your knees, feet and ankles. Avid runners will disagree with me, but when I look at a long-distance runner's physique compared to a sprinter I know which one I would rather have. Long distance endurance training also teaches your body to use energy more efficiently, leading to fat stores. Sprinters tend to be more muscular and lean, while long distance runners tend to be more thin looking and less muscular.

Since I am a big believer that your transformation can be accomplished <u>at home,</u> I am going to focus more on exercises that require little to no equipment. Don't let this fool you though, this program when performed with strict form and at the right intensity level will be very effective and produce some very significant results.

I will describe the exercises to do in the health club, but they are pretty universal and self-explanatory. If you are working out in the club now, I am sure you have a general knowledge of the exercises. If you have questions about proper form, ask the fitness pro at your health club to help you with the exercises. Pick the person that looks most like you want to, and if you are a female that wants to lose body fat and define your muscles, don't ask the 300 pound male power lifter what to do.

If you are going to work-out in the home, here are some guidelines I suggest you follow or you will never accomplish your goals.

KEYS TO THE HOME WORKOUT

1. Find a spot in the house that can be totally set aside for your workout. This area should be free of clutter and only be used to exercise. It does not have to be a large area, just enough so you have room to move freely.

2. Invest in a general purpose bench, a jump rope, a step and the appropriate dumbbells. These items are very inexpensive. You can purchase a weight bench or step second hand for $20, and dumbbells cost about 25 cents a pound. That's only $5 for a 20 lb. dumbbell at Wal-Mart. If you are on a tight budget you can use milk-jugs filled with water and sand for weights and a sturdy coffee table or an adjustable step for a bench. This is all that you need!

3. Make sure the room is properly ventilated and cool.

4. No distractions. During your 30 minutes or less, do not let anything distract you from your workout. If family is around, tell them the house better be on fire to disturb you. Let the machine answer your phone calls, and put a note on your door that says "Back in 30 minutes." If you have young children, plan your workouts when they are napping or at school.

5. Grab a bottle of water, put on some tunes and get ready to Evolve your life!

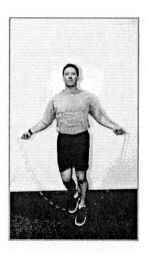

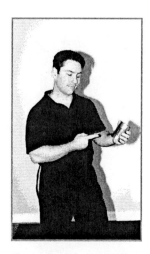

Jumping rope is an excellent workout that requires minimal resources.

If you don't have weights, use a soup can or milk jug.

HOME OR OFFICE WORKOUT

PHASE I– THE EASE IN PHASE

The first phase is designed to let your body slowly and properly adapt to your new exercise program. Several different exercises are performed with fewer sets. This will help you not only learn each movement, but will also help prevent boredom and painful muscle soreness that can occur during the first couple weeks of working-out. Many people quit weight training after a week because they push themselves so hard when they first start that they hurt themselves. That is why it is so important to ease-in. After a couple weeks you will be ready to start pushing yourself. Be patient.

PHASE I– EASE IN   *(2-4 weeks)*

3 days per week / total body workout

See accompanying photo section for exercise examples

Warm-Up

If you have access to a treadmill, do 10 minutes @ 2-4 mph with a 2-4 incline.

If not and weather permits, warm-up outside wtih a brisk walk for 10 minutes.

Another option is to step-ups in your home for 10 minutes.

Stretch

Overall Body Stretch

(Quads, Hams, Upper Back, Lower Back, Chest, Triceps, Biceps, Shoulders, Neck Forearms, Abs)

Day 1

Squat	1 x 25 warm-up
	2 x 20
Good Morning	1 x 20
Step-Ups	1 x 20 each leg
Calf Raise	1 set w/ feet together
	1 set w/ each leg
Chair Lift	2 x 5-10
Reverse Hyper-extension	1 x 5-10
Push-Ups	2 x 10-25
Flys	1 x 10-15

Day 1 Continued

Chair Dip	2 x 10-25
Kickback	1 x 10-15 each side
Broomstick Curl	2 x 10-15
Hammer Curl	1 x 10-15 each arm
Shoulder Press	2 x 10-25
Front Raise	1 x 10-15
Side Raise	1 x 10-15
Abdominal Crunch	2 x 10-25

Day 2

Cardio Only Day

Day 3

Same As Day 1

Day 4

OFF

Day 5

Cardio Only

Day 6

Same as Day 1

Day 7

OFF

CARDIO

If you are doing your cardio separately from your resistance work, cool-down by riding the bike or walking at a leisurely pace for 5 minutes.

If you are doing your cardio at the same time, walk for 20-40 minutes at a leisurely pace or step up and down on a stair or your step at a good pace for 25 minutes. Music or television makes this much easier!

The more cardio you do the faster you will lose fat. If you are on a tight schedule, make sure you are doing at least 3 sessions of Cardiovascular training a week, <u>minimum</u>! These are fat-burning sessions so they are not that hard. If you have a treadmill you can put your TV right in front of it and walk during your favorite shows.

PHASE II– THE MUSCLE BUILD PHASE

Phase II is designed to focus on building new muscle. No more than two muscle groups will be trained on the same day. During this phase you should concentrate on using heavier resistance and fewer reps. By following this method, you will be able to work a specific muscle group harder and allow it to rest longer. This type of training results in accelerated muscle growth and increased strength.

PHASE II– MUSCLE BUILD   (2-4 weeks)

See accompanying photo section for exercise examples

Day 1 (Back)

Warm-Up with Bent over Row	1 x 25
2 Chair Body Lift	2 x 10-15
Bent-Over Row	2 x 10-15
1 Arm Row	1 x 10-15
Reverse Hyper-extension	2 x 8-10
Shrug	2 x 10-20

Day 2 (Chest & Shoulders)

Chest

Warm-Up with shoulder circles and knee push-ups

Flat Wide Push-Up	2 x 10-15
Feet up Push-Up	2 x 10-15
Chair Dips	2 x 10-15
Flys	2 x 10-15

Shoulders

1 minute shoulder circles warm-up

Seated Shoulder Press	2 x 10-15
Front Raise	2 x 10-15
Side Raise	2 x 10-15
Cool Down	

Day 3 (Abs & HIIT)

20-40 minute HIIT session

Abdominal Crunches	2 x 25
Leg Lifts	2 x 25

Day 4 (Arms: Biceps & Triceps)

Warm-Up with alternating curls 1 set of 20 reps each arm

Biceps

Bar or Pole Curls	2 x 10-15
Alternating Curls	2 x 10-15 each
Hammer Curls	2 x 10-15

Triceps

Chair Dip	2 x 10-20
Kick-backs	2 x 10-15 each
Overhead extension	2 x 10-15

Day 5 (Legs)

Warm-up with squats	1 x 25 no weight
Squats	3 x 15-20
Lunges	2 x 10-15 each leg
Step-up	2 x 10-15 each leg
Calf Raises	1 x 25 both legs
	1 x 15-20 each leg

Day 6

OFF

Day 7 (Abs & HIIT Session)

Sprint, Run, or Jog up stairs. Walk Down.		30 min.
Ab crunches	2 x 15-25	
Leg Lift	2 x 15-20	

PHASE III– HIIT / PROBLEM AREAS (2 weeks)

During this phase I recommend focusing on your problem areas. If you are lacking in muscle development repeat Phase II and shorten your rests between exercises. Thirty second breaks should be fine. If you are lacking muscular strength and size repeat Phase II and increase your weight and intensity.

If you are still holding a lot of body fat, follow the following program. Complete the entire workout without resting.

PHASE III– PROBLEM AREAS   (2-4 weeks)

See accompanying photo section for exercise examples

Day 1 (Upper Body)

Pole Lift (Pull-Up)	1 x failure
Step or Jump Rope	30 seconds
Push-ups	1 x failure
Step or Jump Rope	30 seconds
Close-In Push-up	1 x failure
Step or Jump Rope	30 seconds
Hammer Curl	1 x failure
Step or Jump Rope	30 seconds
Front to Side Shoulder Raise	1 x failure
Step or Jump Rope	30 seconds

Day 2 (Lower Body)

Squat	1 x 25
Lunge	1 x 12 each side
Good Morning	1 x 25
Step-up	1 x 25
Calf Raise	1 x 25 each leg

Day 3

OFF

Day 4 (HIIT / Abs)

HIIT Session	30 minutes
Ab Crunches	3 x 25
Leg Raises	2 x 25

Day 5

Repeat Day 1

Day 6

Repeat Day 2

Day 7

Repeat Day 4

PHASE IV– LEAN PHASE

During this phase you will begin to focus on shedding stored body fat. You are in the home stretch right now and you need to kick it up a notch. Your resistance work-outs will be easier and less frequent, but you will have to increase the time you spend doing cardio.

PHASE IV– LEAN PHASE   (2-4 weeks)

See accompanying photo section for exercise examples

Day 1 (Total Body Work-out)

Lower Body

Warm-up with Squats	1 x 25-30
Squat	1 x 20
Step or Jump Rope	30 seconds
Lunge	1 x 15
Step or Jump Rope	30 seconds
Step-up	1 x 15
Step or Jump Rope	30 seconds
Calf Raise	1 x 25 each leg

REST 3 MINUTES

Upper Body

Warm-up with push-ups	10-20
Pull-up or pole lift	1 x max
Reverse Hyper extensions	1 x 15
Step or Jump Rope	30 seconds
Flat Dumbbell Press & Fly	1 x 15 of each
Step or Jump Rope	30 seconds
Close in Push-up	1 x 15
Step or Jump Rope	30 seconds
Alternating Curl	1 x 15

Step or Jump Rope	30 seconds
Shoulder Press	1 x 15
Step or Jump Rope	30 seconds
Trap Raise	1 x 15

Day 2

OFF

Day 3

HIIT/Abs

Day 4

Repeat Day 1

Day 5

HIIT/Abs

Day 6

Rest

Day 7

HIIT/Abs

I strongly suggest during the final phase to get in as many low-impact cardiovascular sessions as possible. You will receive optimal results if you perform 30-45 minutes of biking or walking each morning when you get up, and before you eat. I understand that this is taking up more time than you may currently have, but I guarantee that if you really <u>want</u> to change, you will find the time.

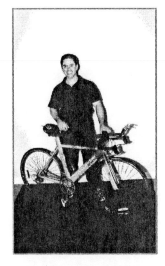

Cycling is an excellent way to have fun while getting fit.

ABBREVIATED TRAINING

As I promised earlier I am including the following shortened workout for those times when you just don't have time. If done properly this training WILL whip you into shape, but you gotta push hard!

ABBREVIATED TRAINING   (8 weeks)

See accompanying photos for exercise examples
Rest 30 seconds between sets and 1 min. between exercises

Day 1

Squat	1 x 15-25 (warm-up)
	3 x 15-25
Lunge	4 x 15 each side
Good Morning	3 x 15
Step-up	3 x 15
Toe Raise (Calf Raise)	1 x 15 (each leg)
	2 x 25 (both together)

Day 2

Warm up with a set of push-ups or knee push-ups

One Arm Row	3 x 15 each arm
Chest Press	4 x 15
Bicep Curl	3 x 15
Shoulder Press	3 x 15
Push ups	4 x max

*You should feel tired between sets, if you are not, you need to push
yourself a little more, by increasing the weight or the reps. To add a
little more kick to your training, jump rope or jog in place for 30
seconds between sets.*

Day 3

Abdominal Crunches	4 x 25-50
Low Impact Cardio	30-60 min.

Day 4

Repeat Day 1

Day 5

Repeat Day 2

Day 6

Repeat Day 3

Day 7

Off

Remember the more often you do HIIT sessions and cardio training, the more body-fat you will burn. I suggest 3x's per week minimum for aerobic training to get better results. It may be hard at first, but you will get used to it in a hurry, and you will feel great when you are done.

Do the above work-out for 8 weeks and you will see a dramatic change in the way you look and feel.

FITNESS CLUB OR HOME GYM

The following workouts follow the same format as the home or office workouts, only they use weights and equipment found in a health club. I'll go through the same phase descriptions for reference, but if you've already read them you can skip to the good part, and start your workout!

PHASE I– THE EASE IN PHASE

The first phase is designed to let your body slowly and properly adapt to your new exercise program. Several different exercises are performed with fewer sets. This will help you not only learn each movement, but will also help prevent boredom and painful muscle soreness that can occur during the first couple weeks of working-out. Many people quit weight training after a week because they push themselves so hard when they first start that they hurt themselves. That is why it is so important to ease-in. After a couple weeks you will be ready to start pushing yourself. Be patient.

PHASE I– EASE IN   *(2-4 weeks)*

See accompanying photo section for exercise examples

Warm-Up

On the treadmill do 10 minutes @ 2-4 mph with a 2-4 incline.

Stretch

Overall Body Stretch

(Quads, Hams, Upper Back, Lower Back, Chest, Triceps, Biceps, Shoulders, Neck Forearms, Abs)

Day 1

Lower Body

Ball Squat	1 x 15-25 (warm-up)
	1 x 15-25
Leg Curl	1 x 15-20
Calf Raise	1 x 10-25
Ab Crunches	10-25 (2-3 sets)

Upper Body

Pull down (wide grip)	1 x 15-25 (warm-up)
Incline Dumbbell Press	1 x 12-15
Reverse & Regular Push Down	1 x 10-15 each
Dumbbell Curls	1 x 10-15 each
Shoulder Front & Side Raise	1 x 10-15 each

Day 2

Cardio

Day 3

OFF

Day 4

Repeat Day 1

Day 5

Cardio

Day 6

Repeat Day 1

Day 7

OFF

CARDIO

If you are doing your cardio separately from your resistance work, cool-down by riding the bike or walking at a leisurely pace for 5 minutes.

If you are doing your cardio at the same time, walk for 20-40 minutes at a leisurely pace or step up and down on a stair or your step at a good pace for 25 minutes. Music or television makes this much easier!

The more cardio you do the faster you will lose fat. If you are on a tight schedule, make sure you are doing at least 3 sessions of Cardiovascular training a week, minimum! These are fat-burning sessions so they are not that hard. If you have a treadmill you can put your TV right in front of it and walk during your favorite shows.

PHASE II– THE MUSCLE BUILD PHASE

Phase II is designed to focus on building new muscle. No more than two muscle groups will be trained on the same day. During this phase you should concentrate on using heavier resistance and fewer reps. By following this method, you will be able to work a specific muscle group harder and allow it to rest longer. This type of training results in accelerated muscle growth and increased strength.

PHASE II– MUSCLE BUILD   (2-4 weeks)

See accompanying photo section for exercise examples

Day 1 (Back)

LAT Pull-down	2 x 8-10
Reverse Hyper-extension	2 x 10
Barbell Row	2 x 10
Pull-ups*	3 x max
Chin-Up	2 x max
Trap Raise to Chin	2 x max

It helps to have a spotter to assist you with your pull-ups

Day 2 (Chest & Shoulders)

Warm-up with chest stretch & shoulder stretch

Shoulder Circles	30 seconds
Push-ups	1 x max
	(use knees if difficult)
Incline Dumbbell Press	2 x 8-12
Dumbbell Fly	2 x 8-12
Shoulder Press	2 x 8-12
Shoulder Side Raise	1 x 15
Shoulder Front Raise	1 x 15
Push-up	1 x max

Day 3 (HIIT/Abs)

HIIT Session	30 minutes
5 minute warm-up	3 mph on treadmill
HIIT Session	1 min walk @ 3.5 mph
	30 second fast run
	repeat for 20 minutes
Cool Down	5 minutes @ 3 mph

Running up hills and walking down is a great HIIT session and running up stairs and walking down is another great option.

Ab Crunches	3 x 25
Leg Raise	1 x 25

Day 4 (Arms: Biceps and Triceps)

Warm-up with Bicep and Tricep stretches

Dumbbell Curls	1 x 15-20 light weight
Kickbacks	1 x 15-20 light weight
Barbell Curls	2 x max
Close Grip Bench	2 x max
Alternate Dumbbell Curls	2 x max
V- Bar Pushdown	2 x max
EZ Curls	1 x max (out grip)
	1 x max (in grip)

Day 5 (Legs)

Warm-up with Quadriceps and Hamstring stretches

Ball Squats	1 x 20-25
Squat	3 x 6-8
Dumbbell Lunge	3 x 6-8
Leg Curl	3 x 8

Day 6

OFF

Day 7 (HIIT/Abs)

Leg Lifts	3 x 25
Ab Crunches	1 x 25

This is the hardest phase. Most of your growth will occur during this type of training. Be sure to stretch properly before, during and after your training. This will prevent injury, increase flexibility and reduce the effects of pain.

PHASE III– HIIT / PROBLEM AREAS (2 weeks)

During this phase I recommend focusing on your problem areas. If you are lacking in muscle development repeat Phase II and shorten your rests between exercises. Thirty second breaks should be fine. If you are lacking muscular strength and size repeat Phase II and increase your weight and intensity. If you are still holding a lot of body fat, follow the following program.

PHASE III– HIIT / PROBLEM AREAS   *(2-4 weeks)*

See accompanying photo section for exercise examples

Day 1 (Upper Body)

LAT Pull-down	1 x failure
Step or Jump Rope	30 seconds
Flat Dumbbell Chest Press	1 x failure
Step or Jump Rope	30 seconds
Close Grip Bench	1 x failure
Step or Jump Rope	30 seconds
Hammer Curl	1 x failure
Step or Jump Rope	30 seconds
Front to Side Shoulder Raise	1 x failure
Step or Jump Rope	30 seconds

Day 3 (HIIT/Abs)

Squat	2 x failure
Lunge	2 x failure
Good Morning	3 x 25
Leg Curl	1 x failure
Calf Raise	2 x failure

Day 3

OFF

Day 4 (HIIT/Abs)

HIIT Session	30 minutes
Ab Crunches	3 x 25
Leg Raises	2 x 25

Day 5

Repeat Day 1

Day 6

Repeat Day 2

Day 7

Repeat Day 4

This phase might seem like a lot of work but none of these work-outs should take anymore than 30 minutes with warm-up and cool-down included. On your lower body day, take no more than 30 seconds of rest. Taking these exercises to failure just means that you cannot do one more repetition with proper form or without the aid of a spotter.

Remember, this is for optimal results. If you begin to feel dizzy or light-headed, take a breather! Really focus on your HIIT sessions. They are very effective for burning fat while retaining valuable muscle. A major mistake that most people make is that they fail to train with the proper intensity. You will learn to love this type of work-out because first of all, it works and secondly, you are not spending hours in the gym; get in and get out! Always train with a sense of urgency.

PHASE IV– LEAN PHASE

During this phase you will begin to focus on shedding stored body fat. You are in the home stretch right now and you need to kick it up a notch. Your resistance work-outs will be easier and less frequent, but you will have to increase the time you spend doing cardio.

PHASE IV– LEAN PHASE   (2-4 weeks)

See accompanying photo section for exercise examples

Day 1 (Total Body Workouts)

Lower Body

Ball Squats	1 x 25-30 (warm-up)
Bench Squat	1 x 20
Lunge	1 x 15
Step-up / Jump Rope	30 seconds
Calf Raise	1 x 15

REST 2 MINUTES

Upper Body

Pull-downs	25 light weight
Pull-ups w/spotter	1 x max
Reverse Hyper-extensions	1 x 15
Step-up / Jump Rope	30 seconds
Flat Dumbbell Press & Fly	1 x 15 each
Step-up / Jump Rope	30 seconds
Close Grip Bench	1 x 15
Step-up / Jump Rope	30 seconds
Barbell Curl	1 x 15
Step-up / Jump Rope	30 seconds
Shoulder Press	1 x 15
Step-up / Jump Rope	30 seconds
Trap Raise	1 x 15

Day 2

OFF

Day 3

HIIT/Abs

Day 4

Repeat Day 1

Day 5

HIIT/Abs

Day 6

Repeat Day 1

Day 7

HIIT/Abs

I strongly suggest during the Final Phase to get in as many low-impact cardiovascular sessions as possible. You will receive optimal results if you perform 30-45 minutes of biking or walking each morning when you get up, and before you eat. I understand that this is taking up more time than you may currently have, but I guarantee that if you really <u>want</u> to change, you will find the time.

ABBREVIATED TRAINING

As I promised earlier I am including the following shortened workout for those times when you just don't have time. If done properly this training WILL whip you into shape, but you gotta push hard!

ABBREVIATED TRAINING   *(8 weeks)*

See accompanying photos for exercise examples
Rest 60 seconds between sets and 2 min. between exercises

Day 1

Squat	1 x 15-25 light weight
	3 x 15-25
Lunge	4 x 15 each side
Good Morning or	3 x 15 each side
Hamstring Curl	
Step-up	3 x 15
Calf Raise	1 x 15 each leg
	2 x 25 both legs

Day 2

Push-ups or Knee Push-ups	1 set (warm-up)
Pull Downs	6 x 15 (3 each arm)
Chest Press	4 x 15
Bicep Curl	3 x 15
Shoulder Press	3 x 15
Push-ups	4 x max

Day 3 (Abs/Cardio)

Abdominal Crunches	4 x 10 max
Low Impact Cardio	30-60 minutes

Day 4

Repeat Day 1

Day 5

Repeat Day 2

Day 6

Repeat Day 3

Day 7

OFF

You should feel tired between sets, if you are not, you need to push yourself a little more, by increasing the weight or the reps. To add a little more kick to your training, jump rope or jog in place for 30 seconds between sets.

Remember the more often you do HIIT sessions and Cardio training, the more body-fat you will burn. I suggest 3x's per week minimum for aerobic training to get better results. It may be hard at first, but you will get used to it in a hurry, and you will feel great when you are done.

Do the above work-out for 8 weeks and you will see a dramatic change in the way you look and feel.

MIX IT UP A BIT!

As you work your way through each phase, there are different levels that you can try in order to vary the level of difficulty in your workouts. If a phase starts to get easier for you to handle, try bumping up to the next level to push yourself. The levels are listed below:

Level 1

Rest 30 seconds between sets and 60 seconds between exercises

Level 2

Rest 30 seconds between sets and no rest between exercises

Level 3

Do 2 sets of each exercise with 30 seconds rest between sets and exercises.

Level 4

Do 2 sets of each exercise with 30 seconds rest between sets and no rest between exercises.

CHAPTER 7

STAYING ON TRACK

One of the main reasons that people fail to become fit is they have difficulty staying on track. Anyone can do anything for a short period of time. The problem with that is, usually that period is so short that it is impossible to become a life changing habit.

My program is only a <u>jump-start</u> to a <u>lifestyle</u> change. You cannot complete your transformation and then go back to your same old bad habits and expect to stay healthy. There are going to be times when you feel like quitting or giving up. Whether it is your body rejecting your dramatic change initially or societal temptation you must have a way to continue your fit lifestyle. Once you have developed healthy habits into a lifestyle it becomes much easier, but you will always face moments of weakness.

I have listed on the following pages some pointers and mental exercises to keep you going strong, keep you getting fitter, and helping you stay on track and evolve your life.

POSITIVE AFFIRMATIONS, RELAXATION, & VISUALIZATION TECHNIQUE

Use your visualization technique again to remind yourself of how good you are going to look. Picture yourself playing with your grand kids or getting back on the basketball court. Really spend some time and concentrate on your long-term goals and all the benefits you will get from sticking with it.

POSITIVE SELF-TALK

This works. Tell yourself over and over that you <u>can</u> and <u>will</u> do it. Tell yourself that you feel stronger and want to be better. Tell yourself that you want to do this for your family, friends and yourself.

READ YOUR LETTER TO YOURSELF

Remember that letter I told you to write? Go back to it. Read through it, take it seriously. See how you have changed.

WRITE A NEW LETTER

Write a new letter to yourself. If you have been training for 2 weeks, write down how you feel compared to when you started. Write down any new reasons for continuing on. Write down how great you feel when you have enjoyed the feeling of discipline and accomplishment.

LOOK THROUGH YOUR JOURNAL

Go back through your journal. Ask yourself if you really want to give up all that hard work you have put behind you. Analyze how much you have improved. Have a feeling of pride in what you have already accomplished. Realize that if you quit now, all that time and work was for nothing.

LOOK AT PICTURES OF FIT PEOPLE

It sounds funny but it is a great motivator. Look at the people that you dream of looking like. This will really motivate you. Do you really think that that cover model is actually mentally stronger than you? No way! If they can do it, I promise you can too!

REMIND YOURSELF THAT YOU CAN ACCOMPLISH ANYTHING!

Look at other things you have done in your life outside of fitness. Whether it be starting a business, graduating from college, raising children, or whatever. All of those things are much harder than staying fit. I always am amazed at all the brilliant and successful people that I know that are out of shape!

USE YOUR NEGATIVE THOUGHT REINFORCEMENT

Some people think that negative thought reinforcement is ineffective. It works great when you need to light a little fire under your butt. Get mad at the fact you try to cover up some parts of your body, get mad that the girl down the street that looks great in a bathing suit and you don't... better yet, get mad that you become out of breath when you take the stairs, get mad that your son can beat you in basketball now. Visualize sitting in that wheelchair when you are older. Imagine not being able to play golf.

LOOK AT YOUR BEFORE PICTURES

Before pictures are a great motivator. Pull them out and look at them. Remind yourself why you don't want to be that person anymore. Take a good long look too! Keep a copy in your wallet or purse. When you feel like quitting pull them out. I can tell you one thing, when you have finished your transformation you can't wait for an opportunity to pull the old ones out to show others what you used to look like.

FIND A PARTNER

If all else fails, find a partner. Someone that has the same goals as you do is perfect. Everyone has a friend or family member that needs to transform. Make it competitive. Challenge each other. Sign a pact to motivate each other. Make a bet to see who does the best. When one of you feels down the other can be supportive. When one doesn't feel like working out the other can pump you up. Also, there is nothing like being able to hang out with someone that is going through the same thing.

Remember, it is alright to slip-up every once in a while, just do not make a habit of it. Slip ups should be followed by a longer stretch of discipline. Nobody ever blew an entire regimen it in one day.

Workout with a partner and hold each other accountable by pushing each other!

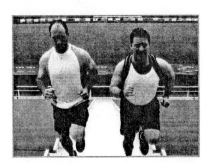

CHAPTER 8

TAKING IT TO THE NEXT LEVEL

For ultimate results I am going to list some things that will not only have a positive effect on your life initially, but will make the transformation process much more dramatic and require less time. Be sure and do these following things along with your regular work-outs and you will achieve even greater results.

1) DO A LOW-IMPACT CARDIOVASCULAR SESSION AS SOON AS YOU GET UP.

30 minutes of biking or walking as soon as you get up will do a few things. First of all you will feel great when you are done because that exercise will release endorphins into your body, put you in a better mood and make the rest of your day feel great. Secondly you will be burning stored calories on an empty stomach which is very effective.

2) EAT 6-8 SMALL MEALS PER DAY.

I have already gone into the importance of eating small meals throughout the day. If you eat every two hours, good healthy meals, you will never have daytime sleepiness or have difficulty waking up in the morning. It will fire up your metabolism and make you a lean machine. You will never be hungry or feel stuffed. Something as little as a nutrition bar or an apple with some cottage cheese is good enough. Make this a habit and you will never feel the same again!

3) GET A MINIMUM OF 8 HOURS OF SLEEP

Rest is key! I know with everybody running around constantly doing this and doing that we sometimes do not put that much priority on sleep. This is a big mistake. Sleep is when our bodies heal and our brain rests. By sleeping a minimum of eight hours every night you will feel great and be more efficient during your daily duties. Go to bed the same time every night and get up the same time every morning. Lying in bed watching TV does not count. Lights out at 10:30 may mean you miss your favorite late night show, but that's why you've got a VCR!

4) EASY ON THE ALCOHOL

We all know how bad alcohol is for us but if you really could really see what it does to your body you wouldn't touch it again. Don't get me wrong, a couple glasses of wine with dinner or a few celebratory beers with the buddies is fine. Keep it to a minimum. It stops your muscles from growing, makes you depressed, has nothing but empty calories and can totally hinder all the work you accomplished during your diet and work out the day before and the day after! It is not worth it.

5) SMOKING

Do I even need to go there?

That's it!

CHAPTER 9

ENRICH YOUR LIFE

I would just like to leave you with a view of mine that has helped make my life better. I am going to follow those few short phrases with a list of simple things that I focus on to make my life more fulfilling.

I do not believe that life is supposed to be easy. It is just a series of challenges that must be taken on and overcome. Those who face these challenges head on get more practice at taking on new challenges. Those who discipline themselves to face challenges rather than avoid them, learn to handle them with greater expertise, and a favorable outcome will result. The more time we spend refining our skills the more fulfilling life will be. The more challenges we overcome the greater sense of accomplishment we will feel.

Worrying about what your weaknesses are will stop you from taking advantage of your strengths. FOCUS.

We have all done things we may not be proud of or regret in our lives, but you have to forget about the past and do your best everyday to change for the better. Be sure not to make a habit of doing things that make you feel guilty later. That is our body's natural mechanism for letting us know when we have made a bad decision.

THE LIST

I began making a list of all the little things to do to make the world a better place. Changing the world does start with you, not your neighbor. These suggestions I am going to share with you have been my real transformation and it can be yours too. I love checking them off my list.

- Get rid of your junk (if you don't need it...get rid of it)
- Organize your life (1 room at a time)
- Make a to do list for your life
- Don't Charge it...If you can't pay cash...save up for it.
- Wear sunscreen
- Floss everyday
- Always do your best in everything

- Listen
- Voice your opinion
- Take your time
- PET your pet
- Lose the mental baggage
- Keep it Simple
- Hug your Mom
- Hug your Dad
- Read for 15 minutes everyday about a topic that interests you
- Be happy
- Smile more
- Remember that 90% of what happens to us is because of us
- Be nice to someone that doesn't like you
- Turn off the TV
- Always be honest
- Do something you always wanted to do but never thought you would.
- Don't Complain
- Be Positive
- If there is a job…do it…now!
- Lead by example
- Don't tell your children…show your children.
- Volunteer

- Don't yell…except at a sporting event
- Help someone who doesn't have it as well as you do
- Do something special for your spouse…just because
- Go to church
- Buy a homeless person dinner
- Spend the day with your grandparents
- Push yourself
- Meet your neighbor
- Listen to your kids more
- Take a chance
- Eat at the dinner table with your family
- Don't be afraid to cry
- Compete
- Smile…I know I already said that one but it works great for me.

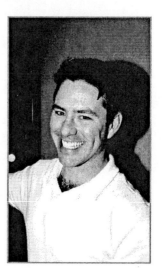

Smiling works for me!

YOU CAN ACCOMPLISH ANYTHING... DON'T FIND REASONS NOT TO OR LET OTHERS TELL YOU, YOU CAN'T! **BECAUSE YOU CAN.**

CHAPTER 10

TASTY, HEALTHY, AND LOW-FAT RECIPES

Use common sense when preparing your meals. Don't starve yourself, instead be sure to snack on healthy fruits and vegetables, this will help you avoid binging on junk!

BREAKFAST

BIG BREAKFAST

- ½ cup cooked oatmeal w/granny smith apple or berries (Mince the apple and cook it with the oatmeal)

- ½ cup egg substitute scrambled in pam w/fresh spinach/ ½ tomato…½ slice cheddar cheese

BREAKFAST BURRITO

- ½ cup egg substitute
- ¼ cup ground turkey
- ½ slice low-fat cheddar cheese
- 1 medium size wheat wrap (cut a big one in half or eat 2 small)

Optional:
- 1 tbsp. red or black beans (about 8 beans)
- 1 tbsp. chunky salsa

Directions:
Brown ground turkey in a skillet/ add egg substitute and cheese. Add salsa. Put filling in wrap.   OR
Wrap in aluminum foil and put in oven.
Heat @ 350° for a few minutes.

BREAKFAST SMOOTHIE

- 1 cup skim milk (cold)
- 1 cup plain LOW-FAT yogurt
- 1 banana
- 1 cup blueberries or strawberries
- 1 serving protein powder

Directions:
Place all ingredients in blender. Push Blend.

SOUPS AND SALADS

BROCCOLI SOUP

- 2 cups chopped broccoli (fresh not frozen)
- 1 cup chicken broth
- 1 cup non-fat evaporated milk
- 2 tsp. canola or olive oil
- Dash of salt and pepper

Directions:

In a large pot cook broccoli in stock for 15 minutes. Pour half the mixture into a blender and puree until smooth. Pour back into the pot and heat, gradually aid milk and oil. Season to taste. Makes 4 servings (70 calories and .65g of fat per serving.)

TURKEY CHILI

- 1lb. low-fat ground turkey
- 1cup diced onion
- 1½ cups diced celery
- 1 diced green pepper
- 5 tsp. chili powder
- 1pt. canned tomatoes
- 1qt. tomato juice
- 1 (6oz) can tomato paste
- 1 (15oz) can chili beans
- 1 (15oz) can kidney beans
- Dash of salt and pepper

Directions:

Brown turkey until ½ done; drain FAT. Add onions and celery. Cook about 15 minutes. Add green pepper and seasonings. Cook about 15 minutes. Pour into large pot and add tomatoes, tomato juice, tomato paste and beans. Simmer 1-2 hours, stirring occasionally. Makes 6 servings (325 calories and 4g of fat)

TOMATO PASTA SOUP

- 1 tsp. olive oil
- ½ cup chopped onion
- 1 clove minced garlic
- 3 lbs. fresh tomatoes, coarsely chopped
- 3 cup fat-free chicken broth
- ½ tsp. basil
- ½ tsp. oregano
- 1 cup uncooked small wheat pasta
- ½ cup fat free mozzarella cheese
- salt and pepper to taste

Directions:

Heat oil in large saucepan over medium heat. Add onion and garlic; cook and stir until onion is tender. Add tomatoes, broth oregano and pepper. Bring to a boil; reduce heat. Cover and simmer 25 minutes. Remove from heat; cool slightly. Puree tomato in blender. Return to saucepan; bring to a boil. Add pasta. Cook pasta 7-9 minutes or until tender. Serve in bowls, sprinkle with cheese. You can substitute 3 cans of whole tomatoes for fresh tomatoes to save time. Makes 8 servings (106 calories and 3g of fat per serving)

CHICKEN SALAD

- ½ cup fat-free salad dressing
- 1 tbsp. dijon mustard
- 4 cup cooked chicken breasts, chopped
- ¼ cup slivered almonds
- ½ cup chopped celery
- dash of salt and pepper

Directions:
Mix ingredients in a bowl. Refrigerate. Makes 6 servings (260 calories and 8g of fat per serving.)

CUCUMBER AND TOMATO SALAD

- 1 cucumber sliced
- 2 chopped tomatoes
- 1 red pepper, chopped
- ¼ sliced red onion
- ¼ cup wine vinegar
- ¼ cup white vinegar
- 1 tbsp. fat-free Italian salad dressing

Directions:
Combine vinegar, Italian dressing. Pour over vegetables. Cover and refrigerate 2 hours. Makes 4 servings (151 calories and NO FAT per serving)

PEPPER TUNA SALAD

- 2 cup thinly sliced zucchini
- ½ cup red bell pepper strips
- ½ cup red bell pepper strips
- ½ cup yellow bell pepper strips
- 1 cup cherry tomatoes, halved
- 1 6oz. can of solid albacore tuna, packed in water, drained
- ¼ cup chopped green onion
- 4 tbsp. fat-free red wine vinegar dressing

Directions:

Pour ¾ cup water into a medium saucepan. Add zucchini and bell pepper strips. Steam veggies about 10 minutes or until crisp tender. Remove from heat; drain any excess water. Place in a serving bowl. Add tomatoes, tuna, and green onions. Coat with dressing, about 4 tablespoons. Makes 4 servings (86 calories and .5g of fat per serving.)

SIDE DISHES & VEGETABLES

OVEN YAM FRIES

- 2 large yams
- olive oil cooking spray
- ¼ tsp. garlic powder
- dash ground pepper

Directions:

Cut yams into ½ inch thick wedges (lengthwise). Place in a large bowl. Generously spray yams with cooking spray and sprinkle with pepper; toss until well coated. In a 400 degree preheated oven place yams on a foil-lined cookie sheet. Bake 35-40 minutes or until tender. Makes 4 servings (65 calories and very little fat per serving)

VEGGIE TRIO

- 1 (10oz.) package frozen green beans
- 1 package frozen broccoli
- 1 package frozen cauliflower
- ½ white onion, sliced
- 1 tbsp. olive oil

Directions:

Cook frozen veggies according to instructions and drain. Heat sauté pan with olive oil on medium high. Place vegetables in heated pan and cook until crispy and bright. Add a dash of salt for taste. Makes 6 servings (Low calories Low FAT)!

BABY EGGPLANT PARMESAN SLICES

- 2 baby eggplants (sliced ½ thick)
- 1 red bell pepper (chopped)
- 2 tbsp. parmesan cheese
- 1 tbsp. olive oil

Directions:

Heat sauté pan on medium high, add olive oil. Add eggplant and pepper. Flip eggplant when golden brown. Put on plate and sprinkle with Parmesan cheese.

MAIN DISHES

Remember: Any combination of lean meat or fish, mixed with some black beans and spinach or broccoli cooked in a heated pan with some olive oil is healthy, tasty and FAST. Take the mixture and spoon it in a wheat wrap with a dollop of salsa and you have a great meal!

PORK TENDERLOIN WITH HERBS

- 2 (1/2 lb.) pork tenderloins
- 2 tsp. olive oil
- 2 cup sliced onions, broken into rings
- 2 garlic cloves, minced
- dash thyme
- dash salt
- dash pepper

Directions:
Preheat oven to 375 degrees. Spray a roasting pan with olive oil. Remove all fat from tenderloin. Slit down center of each tenderloin lengthwise. Do not cut all the way through. Open both tenderloins so they lie flat; place in pan. Add olive oil to large skillet. When oil is hot, cook onions and garlic until tender. Stir in seasoning. Spread onion mixture evenly over tenderloins. Bake in oven for 40 to 50 minutes at 375. Makes 4 servings (180 calories and 6 grams of fat per serving).

CHICKEN QUESADILLAS

- ½ lb. thinly sliced chicken breast
- ½ cup finely chopped onion
- ½ cup finely chopped red or green pepper
- ¼ cup salsa
- 1 cup LOW-FAT Colby and Monterey Jack shredded cheese
- 8 NO-FAT wheat tortillas
- olive oil cooking spray

Directions:

Preheat oven to 450 degrees. Combine onion and pepper in microwave-save bowl; cover with plastic wrap. Pierce with fork and microwave on high 2-3 minutes. Stir in salsa. Sprinkle 2 tablespoons cheese evenly on each tortilla. Arrange chicken over cheese and top with 1 tablespoon salsa. Fold tortillas over to close. Lightly spray 2 baking sheets with cooking spray. Place 4 quesadillas on each sheet. Lightly spray tops with cooking spray. Bake 10 minutes or until lightly browned. Makes 8 servings (175 calories and 5 grams of fat per serving).

TURKEY SAUSAGE AND CHICKEN JAMBALAYA

- ½ lb. turkey sausage (sliced in chunks)
- 2 green peppers, diced
- 3 plum tomatoes
- 1 cup chopped onions
- 2 celery stalks, sliced
- 1 tbsp. minced scallions
- 4 cloves of garlic, minced
- ¼ lb. chicken breasts, cut in 1-inch pieces
- 1 cup reduced-fat chicken broth
- 1.5 cups brown rice
- ½ tsp. hot pepper sauce
- 1 tsp. worcestershire sauce

Directions:

Over medium heat sauté sausage until lightly browned; drain on paper towels. Add peppers, tomatoes, onions, celery, scallions and garlic. Sauté until vegetables are tender. Add chicken and cook for 5 minutes. Stir in sausage, broth, Worcestershire sauce and hot pepper sauce. Cover and simmer until rice is tender, 10 minutes. Makes 4 servings (350 calories and 10 grams of fat per serving.)

FANTASTIC FAJITAS

- 8 wheat tortillas (7")
- 3 turkey or chicken breast cutlets
- 1 red bell pepper
- 1 green bell pepper
- 2 tbsp. salsa
- dash pepper

Directions:

Heat oil in a large skillet over medium-high heat. Slice cutlets and peppers into thin strips. Place strips in skillet, add pepper and salsa, and cook until meat is done. Warm tortillas in the microwave for 30-40 seconds under a slightly damp paper towel. Spoon filling into tortillas, roll-up, and enjoy! Makes 4 servings (300 calories and 8g of fat per serving.)

VEGGIE SUPPER COMBO

- 2 tbsp. olive oil
- ½ cup chopped onion
- ½ cup chopped green bell pepper
- ½ cup chopped red bell pepper
- 1 cup Broccoli
- ½ cup uncooked brown rice
- ½ cup uncooked lentils
- 14 ½ oz low-salt chicken broth
- 1 tbsp. worcestershire sauce
- ¼ tsp. garlic powder
- ¼ tsp. red pepper
- 1 (15oz.) can black-eyed peas, drained

Directions:

Heat oil in a large skillet over medium heat until hot. Add onion, bell pepper, rice and lentils. Cook and stir 3 to 4 minutes or until vegetables are tender. Stir in remaining ingredients. Bring to a boil. Reduce heat to low; cover and simmer 15 to 20 minutes or until vegetables are tender and liquid is absorbed, stirring occasionally. Makes 4 servings (340 calories and 8 grams of fat per serving).

CHICKEN OR FISH & RICE CASSEROLE

- 1 cup cooked, diced chicken breast (8oz.)

OR

- 1cup cooked, chunked white fish (10oz.)

- ½ cup celery, chopped (2 stalks)
- 1 cup broccoli pieces
- 1 cup brown rice
- ½ cup diced onion
- ½ cup sliced mushrooms
- 2 cup salt free chicken broth
- 1 small can low-fat, low-salt cream of mushroom soup

Directions:

Preheat oven to 350 degrees. Mix all ingredients except broccoli; stir well. Bake in covered casserole dish for 45 minutes. Stir in broccoli and bake for another 15 minutes. Leave uncovered for 5 minutes and serve. Make 4 servings (240 calories and 6 grams of fat per serving).

DIPS

HOT CRAB DIP

- 8 oz. no-fat cream cheese, softened
- 8 oz. crab meat
- 1 tbsp. chopped onion
- 1 tsp. horseradish
- dash salt
- ¼ tsp. red pepper
- dash black pepper
- 1 tbsp. skim milk
- 2 squirts worcestershire sauce

Directions:

Preheat oven to 375 degrees. Soften cheese with milk. Blend all ingredients together well. Bake at 375 degrees for 15 minutes or until bubbly. (14 calories per serving and NO-FAT)

CREAM CHEESE SALSA DIP

- 1 (8oz) package fat free cream cheese
- ¼ c. salsa

Directions:

Mix cream cheese and salsa until blended. Serve with veggies. Makes 12 servings (20 calories and NO FAT per serving).

LAYERED MEXICAN DIP

- 1 (8oz.) pkg. fat-free cream cheese, softened
- 1.5 cup no-fat shredded cheddar cheese
- ¼ cup sliced green onion
- 1 garlic clove, minced
- 1 cup salsa
- ½ cup chopped tomato

Directions:

Mix cream cheese, ¼ c. cheddar cheese and 3 tablespoons of the onions and garlic. Spread onto 9-inch pie plate, Mix salsa and tomato; spread over cream cheese mixture. Sprinkle with ¾ cup cheddar cheese and 1 tablespoon onion. Makes 8 servings (69 calories and NO FAT).

DESSERTS

Fruit is always a good choice! Be creative!

SUGAR FREE JELL-O

- with added fruit pieces is great.

GRAHAM CRACKERS & VANILLA WAFERS

- these are alright in moderation

NO-FAT ORANGE WHIPPED CREAM

- ½ cup instant nonfat dry milk
- ½ cup freshly squeezed orange juice

Directions:

Whip dry milk and orange juice until fluffy. Makes 1 cup (25 calories and no fat per tablespoon).

CRANBERRY-BERRY LEMONADE COCKTAIL

- 4 cup sugar free lemonade
- 1 cup cranberry juice
- 1 cup raspberries
- 1 cup soda water

Directions:

In blender combine raspberries and 2 cups lemonade. Blend until smooth. Pour into pitcher. Add remaining ingredients. Stir gently. Serve immediately. Makes 10 (½ cup) servings (70 calories and NO FAT per serving).

BERRY-BANANA SHAKE

- ½ cup skim milk
- ½ cup strawberries, frozen
- ½ cup blueberries, frozen
- ½ cup frozen nonfat vanilla yogurt
- ½ ripe banana, sliced

Directions:

Combine all ingredients in a blender.
Blend until smooth.
Makes 1 serving (250 calories and 1 gram of fat).
If you must eat fast food, these are your best choices:

SMART FAST FOOD CHOICES

If you HAVE to eat fast food, here are some good choices:

Wendy's Mandarin Chicken Salad

Mixed greens, chicken breast, roasted almonds, mandarin orange segments, and half a packet of Oriental sesame dressing make this **420 calorie** salad taste great.

Burger King Chicken Whopper Jr.

Any grilled chicken sandwich is a good choice, but this one actually tastes grilled. The junior size is best -- just because it's a normal-sized sandwich. The junior has **350 calories**, while the regular Chicken Whopper has 580 calories.

Subway's Low-Fat Subs

The new low-fat select subs -- honey mustard ham, sweet onion chicken teriyaki, and red wine vinaigrette club -- range from 310 to 370 calories are "downright delicious."

McDonald's Fruit & Yogurt Parfait

Eat it for breakfast, as a snack, a dessert, or a small lunch. It's two-thirds cup of berries layered between low-fat yogurt and topped with crunchy granola -- all at **380 calories** and 2 grams saturated fat.

Burger King Veggie Burger

It's the first meatless sandwich from a burger chain, with less than two grams saturated fat and fewer calories (330) than just about any hamburger at any chain.

CHECK OUT MY WEBSITE AT

WWW.EVOLVEYOURLIFE.COM

FOR MORE TASTY, HEALTHY RECIPES!

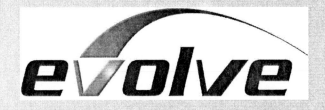

WORKOUT PHOTOS

THE "HOW TO" SECTION OF EXERCISES

STRETCHES

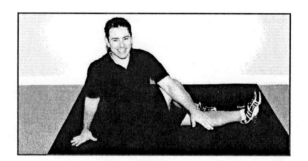

LOW BACK TWIST

Sit on floor with left leg straight out in front. Bend right leg, cross right foot over, place outside left knee. Pull right knee across body toward opposite shoulder. Hold 10 to 20 seconds. Repeat on other side. Breathe easily.

HAMSTRING STRETCH

Sit with the upper body nearly vertical and legs straight. Lean forward using hip flexion and grasp toes with each hand. Slightly pull toes toward the upper body, and pull chest toward the legs. If flexibility is limited, try to grasp the ankles.

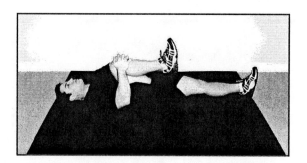

SUPINE KNEE FLEX

From above position, straighten one leg. Pull the other knee into your chest until you feel a stretch in your hip. Switch legs.

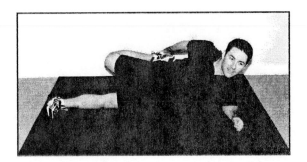

SIDE QUAD STRETCH

Lie down on your side using your elbow for balance. Using other arm, slowly pull your foot towards your butt, keeping both knees together and bent knee pointing down. Switch legs.

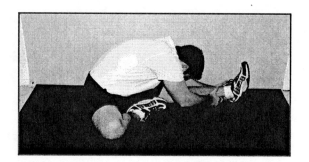

SEMI STRADDLE

Lean forward over your left leg until you feel a stretch behind your knee and in your calf. Hold that position by grasping the left leg. Repeat with the right leg.

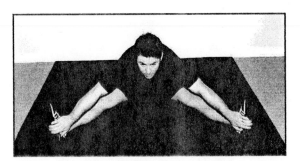

STRADDLE

Sit with the upper body nearly vertical and legs straight. Spread legs as far apart as possible. Grasp toes of each foot and pull slightly. Pull torso forward and toward the ground.

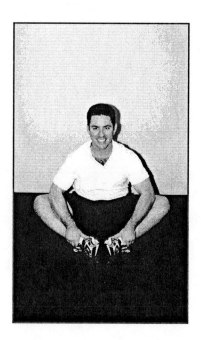

BUTTERFLY

Sit on floor with feet pressed together. Keeping abs in, lean forward until you feel a gentle stretch in your inner thighs.

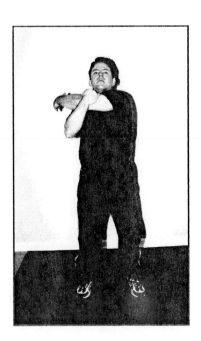

UPPER BACK STRETCH

Stand and place left hand on right shoulder. With right hand, pull left elbow across chest toward right shoulder and hold. Repeat on other side.

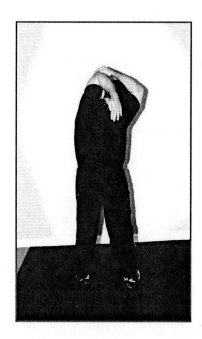

SIDE BEND OBLIQUE STRETCH

Keep knees slightly flexed. Flex left elbow above your head. Reach for your right shoulder blade with your left hand. Grasp the left elbow with the right hand. Pull elbow behind head while keeping elbow bent. Lean from waist to the right side. Repeat with other side.

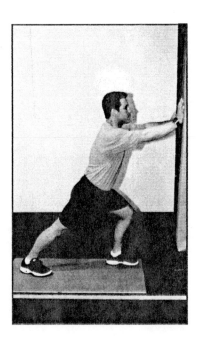

CALF STRETCH

Stand a little way from wall and lean on it with palms. Place left foot in front of you, leg bent, right leg straight behind you. Slowly move hips forward until you feel stretch in calf of right leg. Keep right heel flat and toes pointed straight ahead. Repeat on other side. Do not hold breath.

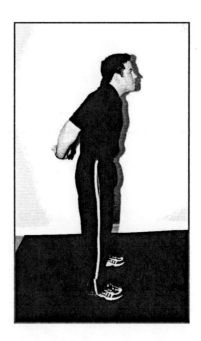

STRAIGHT ARMS BEHIND BACK

Standing, place both arms behind back. Interlock fingers with palms facing each other. Extend elbows fully. Slowly raise the arms, keeping the elbows straight. Keep head upright and neck relaxed.

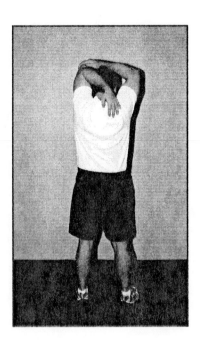

TRICEP STRETCH

Standing, abduct left shoulder and flex the elbow. Grasp right elbow with left hand. Pull elbow behind head with right hand to increase shoulder abduction. Switch arms and repeat on other side.

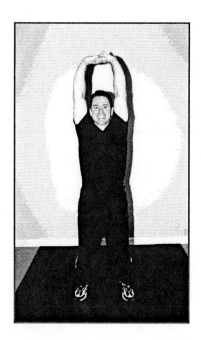

PILLAR STRETCH

Stand with arms in front of torso, fingers interlocked with palms facing out. Slowly straighten arms above head with palms up. Continue to reach upward with hands and arms. While continuing to reach upward, slowly reach slightly backward.

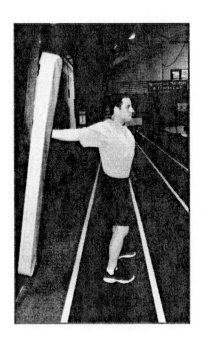

CHEST STRETCH

Place your right palm against a stable object like
a doorway, wall, or support post. Keep your arm
perpendicular, turning your body to the left until you
feel a stretch in your chest muscle. Repeat other side.

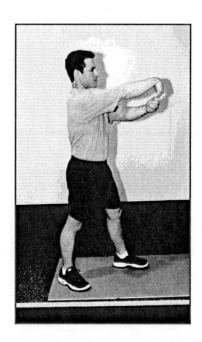

FOREARM STRETCH

Without raising the shoulders, extend the affected arm straight out in front of the body and slowly, gently bend the wrist down with the free hand. Keep the fingers over the knuckles of the bent hand, not over the fingers.

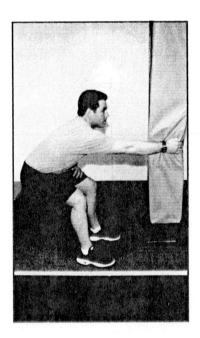

UPPER BACK PULL

Stand tall, feet slightly wider than shoulder-width apart, knees slightly bent. Using one hand, grab the pillar pulling toward you, allowing your upper back to relax. Rest your other hand on your thigh. You should feel the stretch between your shoulder blades.

LEGS/BUTT

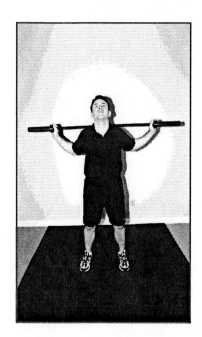 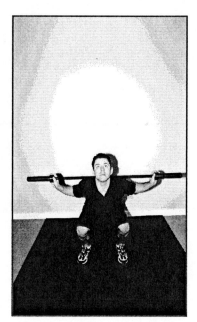

SQUATS

Lift the bar up and place behind your neck. Point your feet <u>straight</u> and bend at the knees bringing the bar down with you. Squat until your thighs are parallel to the ground if possible. As you squat down keep your head up and your back slightly arched.

LEGS/BUTT

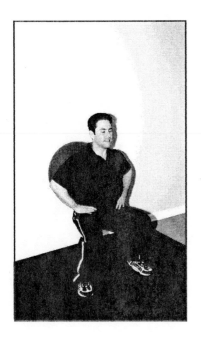 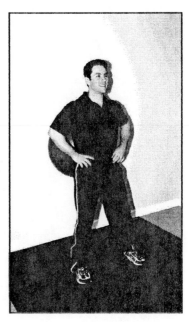

BALL SQUATS

Place a ball on the wall at the level of your lower back. Place the ball so that the curve of the ball is right in the small of your back. Point your feet straight and lean back into ball. Make sure your back is vertical as you do so. Slowly and with control, while pushing back on the ball, squat down until your thighs are parallel to the floor. Pushing back on the ball stand back up, rolling the ball back up the wall.

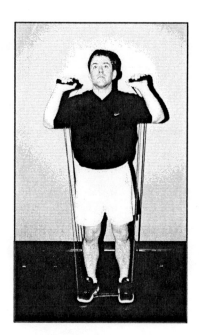 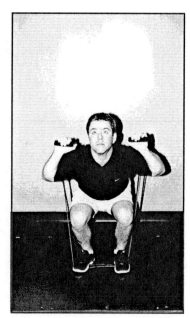

SQUAT WITH CORDS

Same as the squat only using cords. Keep feet shoulder length apart and step on cords placing underneath arch of foot. Point your feet straight and bend at the knees bring the cords down with you. Squat until your rear is at about the level of your knees and stand back up. As you squat down keep your head up and your back arched somewhat.

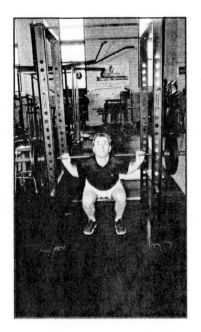 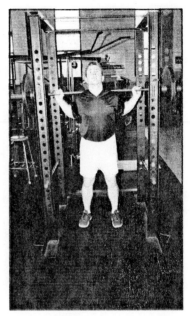

SQUATS

To get into position bring your feet forward and lean back into the bar so that it rests just above your shoulder blades. After you are leaning on the bar bring your pelvis back so that your back is arched. Squat down with the bar until your thighs are parallel to the floor. Extend the legs, standing back up and return to the start position. (**Caution:** Make sure you stay flat footed and do not allow your knees to travel too far in front of your toes.)

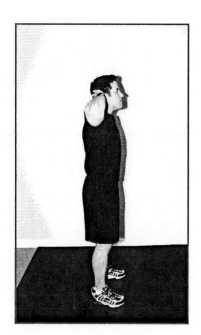 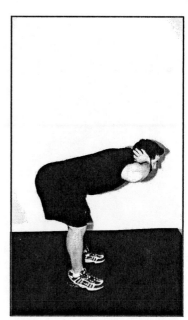

GOOD MORNING

Stand with your feet closer than shoulder width apart. Start straight up keeping your hands behind your ears. Bend at the waist while keeping your back flat and your head up. Once you feel a stretch in the back of your legs, return to the starting position.

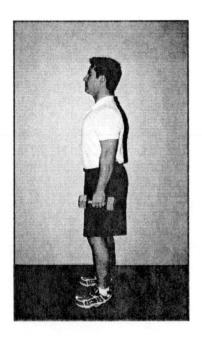 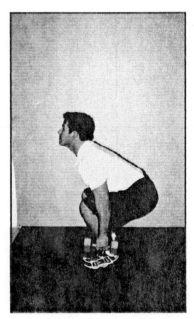

DUMBBELL SQUAT

Hold two dumbbells on either side of your body. Point your feet straight and stand upright. Squat down bringing the dumbbell towards the floor keeping your back flat and knees bent. After going down to parallel, stand back up and repeat.

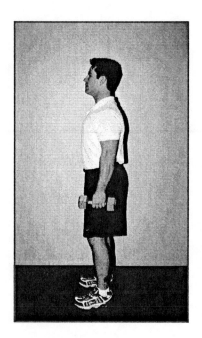 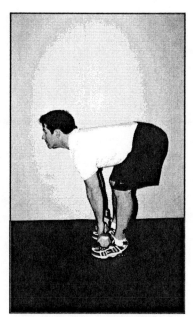

STIFF LEG DEAD LIFT

Start standing upright with a slight lean backwards as shown in the start position. Bend over and as you do so bring your pelvis back as far as you can and extend the arms down and forward as much as you can. Keep the arms completely locked. Once you have come down as far as you can stand back up to the starting position.

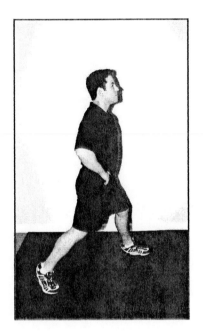 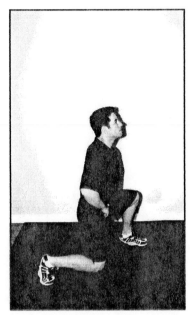

LUNGES

Start by standing upright with your feet together. For beginners place your hand on your hips. Take a long step and bend both knees and lunge towards the floor. Keep you feet pointed straight. It is important to keep the front knee over the heel and not over the toes. In other words if you lunge too far forward you will put great pressure on your front knee and increase the risk of injury. Lower your back knee to the ground, and then push back up with your front foot. Perform required amount of reps, then switch to other side.

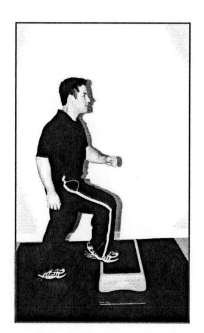 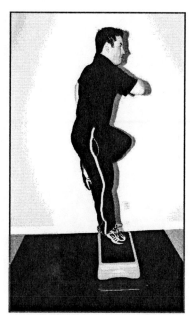

STEP-UPS

Start with your back and shoulders straight and slightly arched, arms bent at the elbows at a ninety degree angle and hands and head pointed straight ahead. Push off with the calves and drive the knee as high as possible as you step up. Repeat switching legs.

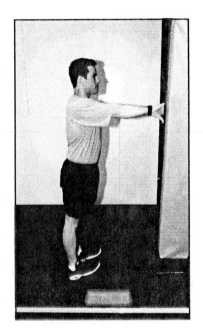 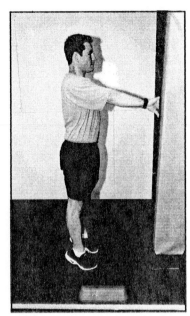

CALF RAISES

Stand on the foot platform on the balls of your feet. Start with your heels as far down below the platform as possible. SLOWLY bring your heels up contracting the calf muscles. Come all the way to the top and hold your contraction on the top for at least 1 second. After 1 second SLOWLY bring your heels back down all the way and repeat.

LEGS/BUTT

BACK

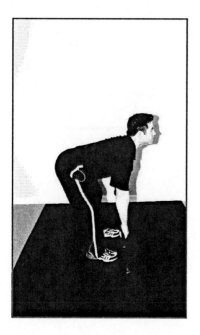 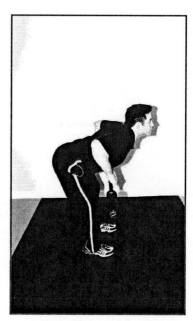

BENT-OVER ROW

Bend your knees and bend your body over so that your back is flat and parallel with the ground. Arch your back and point your toes forward. Pick up the barbell so that is slightly wider than a shoulder width grip. The row motion is pulling the barbell straight up into your mid-section. Pull the barbell right between your upper abdominal muscles and lower chest.

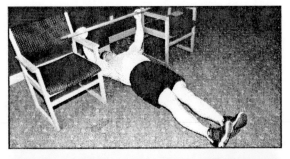

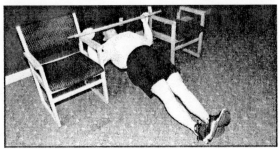

BACK

BROOMSTICK CHAIR PULL

Lie down on the floor. Center you hands on the bar so they are equal distance from the center of the bar.

Lift yourself up toward the bar, to about the middle of your chest. While exhaling lower yourself back down to the starting position.

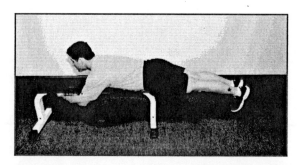

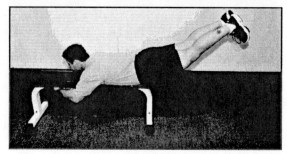

REVERSE HYPER EXTENSIONS

Begin by lying face down on a flat bench with your lower torso hanging off the end of the bench and your feet just short of touching the floor. Grasp under the bench with both hands to support your body. Slowly raise your feet upward until they are just short of parallel with the ground. Then, reverse direction and return your legs to the start position. (An old coffee table can be used, just be sure it is sturdy.)

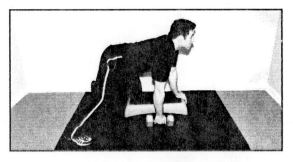

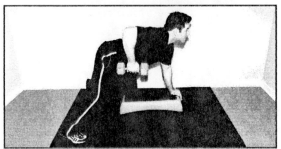

ONE ARM DUMBBELL ROWS

On a bench or step, using your left hand and left knee for stability, flatten your back so that it is parallel with the ground. Grab the weight and raise your elbow until you create a 90° angle with your arm. Return to the start position and repeat.

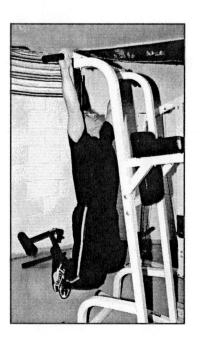 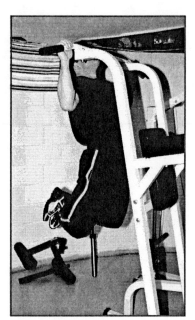

PULL-UPS

An old fashion exercise but very effective. Grab onto the bar and pull your body up until your chin or face is at the level of the bar. Exhale on the way up and inhale on the way down.

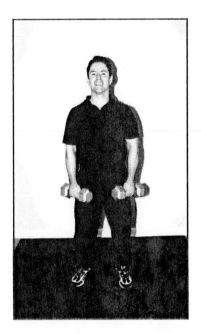 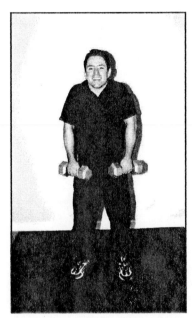

BACK

SHOULDER SHRUGS

Stand up and hold both dumbbells at the sides of your body. Lifting from the shoulder raise the dumbbells as high as you can. Exhale on the way up and inhale on the way back down.

CHEST

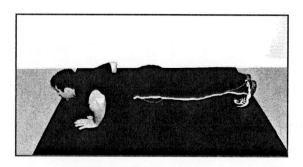

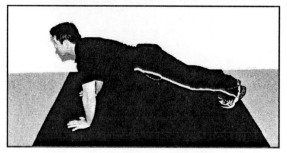

PUSH-UP

This is an oldie but a goodie. Get down on the floor and spread your hands a few inches wider than shoulder width apart. Push off the floor extending your arms and then come back down to the floor. Exhale on the way up and inhale on the way down. (If you have difficulty doing this, rest on your knees instead of your feet.)

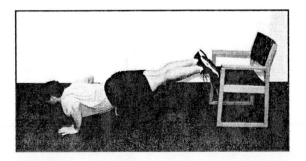

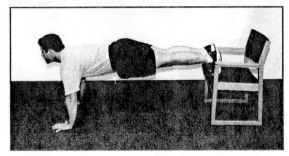

CHEST

CHAIR PUSH-UP

Lying face forward on the floor and a chair behind you, place your legs on top of the chair. Spread your hands a few inches wider than shoulder width apart. Push off the floor extending your arms and then come back down to the floor. Exhale on the way up and inhale on the way down.

CHEST

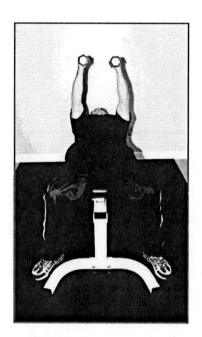 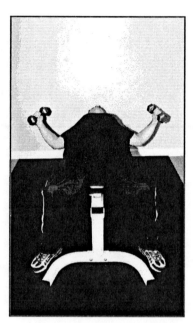

DUMBBELL FLYS

Lie flat on a bench. Start with dumbbells extended over your chest. Bend your elbows slightly while bringing them down even with the bench. Do this without changing the position of your arms.

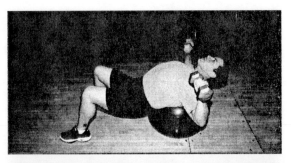

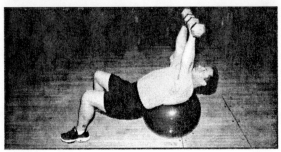

CHEST

DUMBBELL PRESS WITH BALL

Lie down with your back flat on an exercise ball. Take two dumbbells and spread them so that your chest muscles get a good stretch. This will facilitate full range of motion during the exercise. Press the dumbbells straight up and bring them together in the middle, over the mid part of your chest. Bring the dumbbells back down & continue.

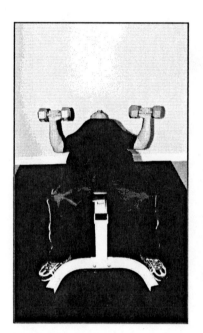 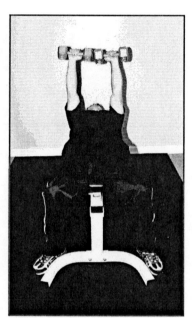

DUMBBELL PRESS

Lie flat on your back on an exercise bench. Hold two dumbbells out to your side so your arms create a 90° angle. Press the dumbbells up. Slowly lower them back to the starting position.

TRICEPS

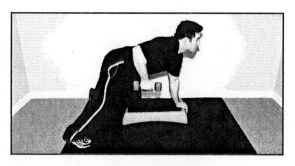

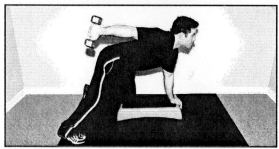

TRICEPS

DUMBBELL KICKBACKS

Rest the left knee and left hand on the bench or step. Bend over so that your back is flat, parallel with the ground. Start with your right arm at a 90° angle. Using the elbow like a hinge of a door, extend the arm towards the back until it is completely straight. Return to starting position & repeat.

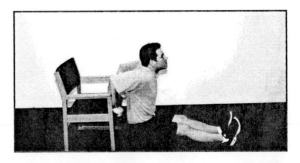

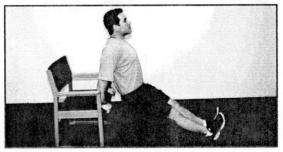

TRICEPS

SINGLE ARMCHAIR DIPS

Place your hands on the edge of a chair. Walk your feet out away from the chair and extend your legs out keeping your feet close together. Slowly bend the elbows and let the body dip down to where your rear is just off the floor. Extend the arms back up to complete the repetition.

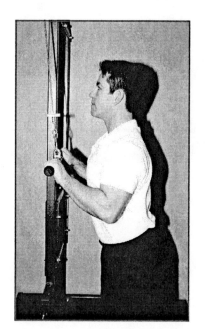 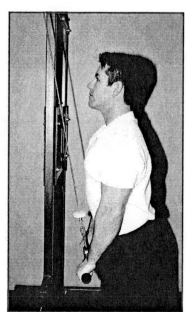

TRICEPS

TRICEP PUSHDOWN

Attach a curl bar to a cable pulley and make sure it is high enough so that you need to reach up to grab it. Place your hands palm down on the bar and bring your elbows forward slightly. Using the elbows as your pivot point push the bar all the way down until the arms are fully extended and then bring the bar back to just above the middle of the chest, being careful not to lift the elbows as you do so.

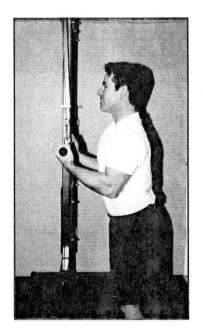 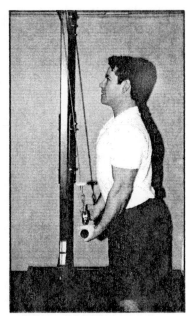

REVERSE TRICEP PUSH DOWN

Adjust a cable pulley machine so that the pulley is high above your head. Attach a bar to the clip. Grab the bar with your hand very close together as shown and your palms up. Bring the elbow down to the side of your body as you begin the exercise and be sure to keep them there. Allowing the handle bar to rotate in your hands pull on the bar, straightening your arms to a full extension. As you do so make sure you keep your wrists straight. Exhale on the way down and inhale on the way up.

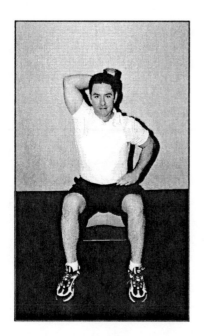 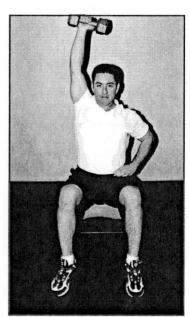

TRICEPS

ONE ARM TRICEP EXTENSION

While sitting, start with a dumbbell behind your head with your elbow bent and forearm parallel to the ground, extend your hand up until the back of your arm is flexed. Repeat with your other arm.

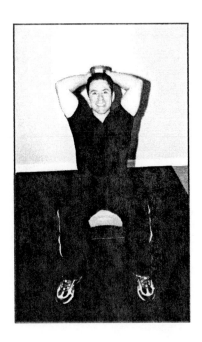 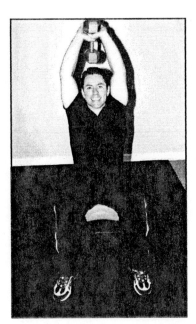

TRICEPS

TWO ARM TRICEP EXTENSION

Sit holding the dumbbell in both hands behind your neck. Inhale and extend your arms straight until they are above your head. It is important to contract your ab muscles to avoid arching your back. Exhale as you complete the movement.

TRICEPS

BICEPS/FOREARMS

BICEPS

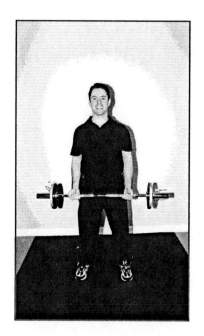 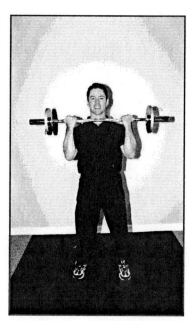

EZ CURL

Stand upright and hold the bar as shown in the start position photo. Start with the arms completely straight curl the bar up, flexing the arms.

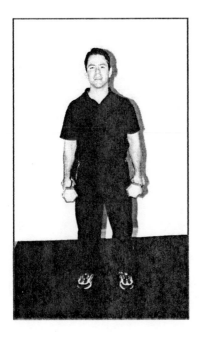 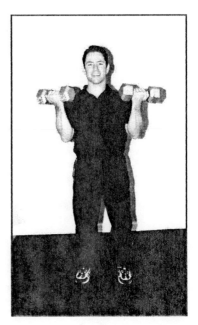

DUMBBELL CURL

Stand upright and hold two dumbbells with the palms up. Bring the elbows forward slightly and begin the exercise with you arms completely straight. Curl the dumbbells all the way up and flex your biceps at the top of the exercise. Return to the start position and repeat.

BICEPS

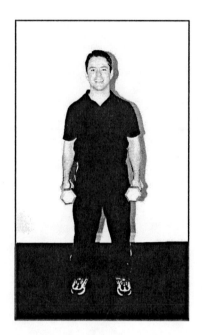 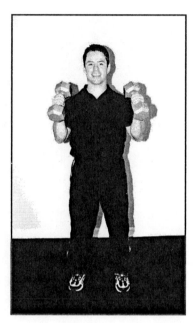

HAMMER CURL

BICEPS

Let your arms hang at your sides. Keeping your elbows in tight, raise the dumbbells to your shoulders. Slowly return to the start position, and repeat.

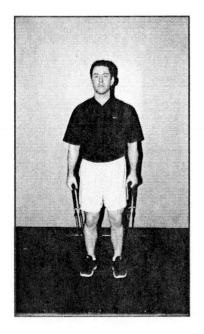 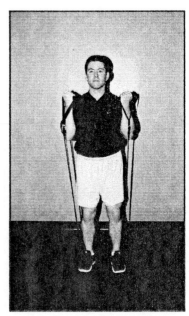

BICEP CURL WITH CORDS

Stand with your feet over the cord. Grab the cords as shown with the palms facing in. Next, curl your biceps and bring your hands up toward your shoulders, twisting your wrists as you clear your legs. Slowly return to the start position and repeat.

BICEPS

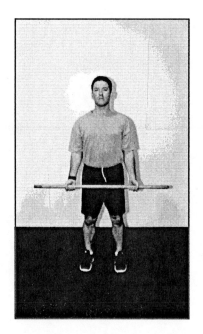 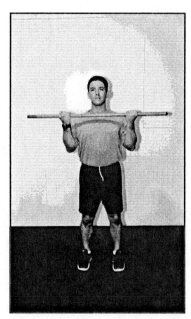

BROOMSTICK CURL

Grab the stick as shown with the palms up. Next, bring your elbows forward and begin the exercise with the arms straight. Curl the stick up, flexing your biceps as you bring towards your shoulders. Slowly lower the broomstick and repeat.

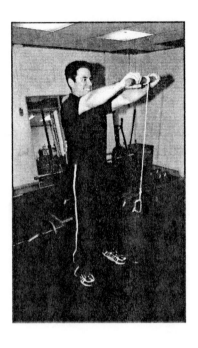

WRIST ROLL

Standing, feet shoulder length apart, take an overhand grip with hands at eye level. Curl your wrists back toward you until the weight is at the top position, then slowly roll back down. (All you need is a 12" piece of pipe, a rope, and some weight to create this piece of equipment.)

BICEPS

BICEPS

SHOULDERS

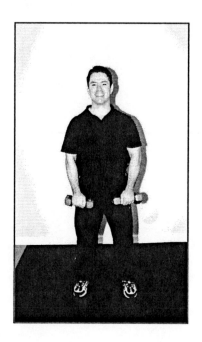 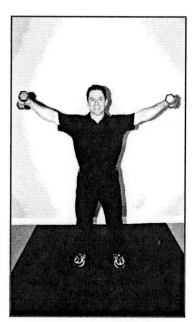

STANDING SIDE RAISES

Stand with your feet slightly spread. Keep your back straight, your arms hanging at your sides, holding one dumbbell in each hand. Raise the dumbbells to the ear level, keeping your elbows slightly bent. Return to the starting position.

SHOULDERS

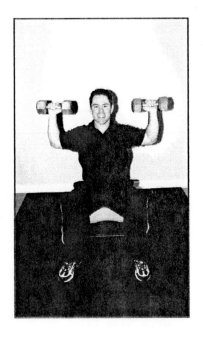 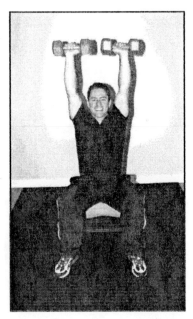

DUMBBELL SHOULDER PRESS

Sit on a step, exercise ball, or bench. Hold two dumbbells at your side with a 90 degree angle in your elbows and the palms facing forward. Press the dumbbells over your head bringing them together at the top.

SHOULDERS

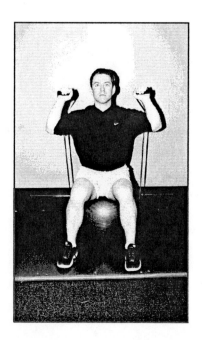 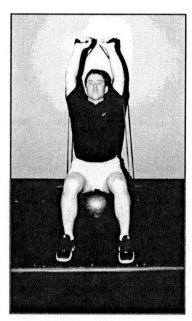

SHOULDER PRESS WITH CORDS

Sit on an exercise ball. Hold the cords to your side with a 90 degree angle in your elbows and the palms facing forward. Press the handles up over your head bringing them together at the top.

SHOULDERS

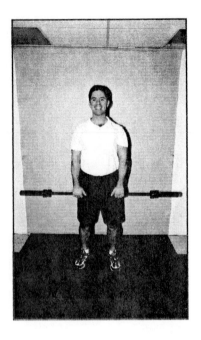
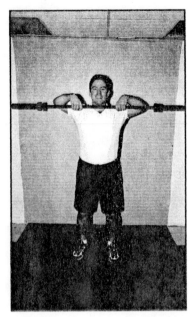

UPRIGHT ROW

Hold the bar in front of you as shown in the start position. Raise the elbows bringing the bar under your chin.

SHOULDERS

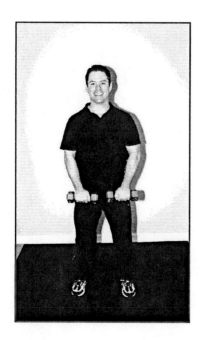 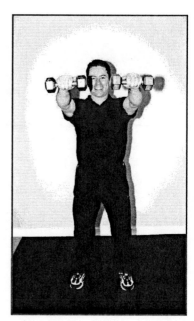

FRONT DUMBBELL RAISES

Hold two dumbbells close together in front of you with your palms facing your body. Using both arms lift the dumbbells directly in front of you until they are at eye level. Slowly lower them to the start position and repeat.

ABS

ABS

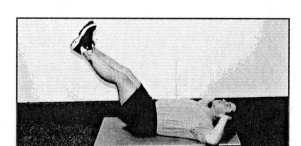

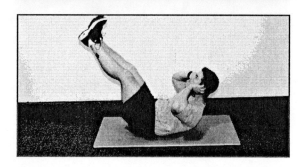

CRUNCHES

Lay down on your back and put your legs up in the air with about a 90 degree angle in your knees. Support your head (not your neck). Curl the upper body up doing a crunch and be sure to keep tension in the abdominal muscles throughout the entire set. Blow air out at the top of the crunch.

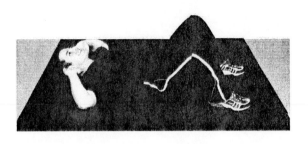

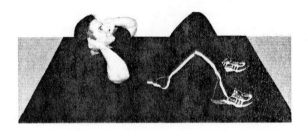

BENT-KNEE CRUNCH

Start at the bottom. Contract the abdominal muscles bringing the upper body up as shown in the finish position.

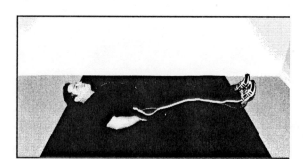

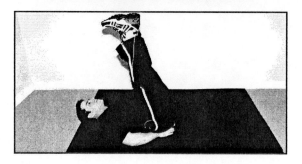

LEG RAISES

Lie on your back on the floor. Cross your feet and lift your legs in the air above you as shown in the finish position. When bringing your legs down, try not to touch the floor.

ABS

This is just the beginning of your Fitness Evolution.

CHECK OUT MY WEBSITE FOR MORE HELPFUL
TIPS, FACTS, AND ANSWERS!

WWW.EVOLVEYOURLIFE.COM

Printed in the United States
15835LVS00006B/61-414